YOUR HEART: AN OWNER'S MANUAL

ARE YOU AT RISK FOR CARDIOVASCULAR DISEASE AND STROKE? Every day, without thinking, millions of Americans set the stage for heart disease, disability, and death. This book will show you how to protect and preserve the most important organ in your body: your heart. Here is the American Heart Association's entertaining yet authoritative owner's manual, essential step-by-step maintenance for everyone of every age. *You can change the odds!* Master the basics and take charge of your heart with the most powerful tools of all—knowledge and motivation:

- Learn the seven risk factors for heart disease
- Track your lifestyle habits
- Begin the six steps to successful lifestyle modification
- Help manage your triggers with strategies that work
- Learn how to get help, set goals, and prevent relapse
- Discover how to eat in or dine out: healthful shopping and cooking hints and heart-healthy choices from any ethnic cuisine or fast-food menu
- Practice heart-healthy travel with the AHA's savvy tips
- Celebrate with party tactics to live for and more!

The Road to Better Health begins with
YOUR HEART: AN OWNER'S MANUAL

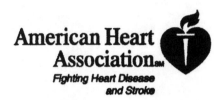

American Heart Association

Fighting Heart Disease and Stroke

Your Heart
An Owner's Manual

American Heart Association's Complete
Guide to Heart Health

POCKET BOOKS
New York   London   Toronto   Sydney

The techniques, suggestions and ideas contained herein are not intended to replace the advice of a physician or trained health professional. If you know or suspect that you have a health problem, you should consult your physician or health professional. The publisher and the American Heart Association disclaim any liability for injury or loss resulting, directly or indirectly, from the use and application of any of the ideas or suggestions contained in this book.

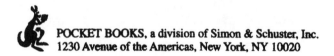

POCKET BOOKS, a division of Simon & Schuster, Inc.
1230 Avenue of the Americas, New York, NY 10020

Copyright © 1995 by American Heart Association

ISBN 978-1-4516-2807-4

First Pocket Books printing March 1996

19 18 17 16 15 14 13 12 11 10

POCKET and colophon are registered trademarks of Simon & Schuster Inc.

Cover art by Marc Galindo/Custom Medical Stock Photo

Printed in the U.S.A.

ACKNOWLEDGMENTS

Your Heart: An Owner's Manual was a labor of love. It was created by a hardworking team, each of whom was on fire with the hope that this project will help people avoid America's number one killer, heart disease.

I want to thank Mary Winston, Ed.D, R.D., AHA Senior Science Consultant, who was the anchor of the team. She tirelessly checked and double-checked the scientific details of the book.

The text, based on American Heart Association materials, was provided by a group of educators and scientists from the Cooper Institute for Aerobics Research in Dallas, Texas. Project director Ruth Ann Carpenter, M.S., R.D., wrote much of the text. She also coordinated the major contributions by Brenda S. Mitchell, Ph.D., and Pamela M. Walker, Ph.D.

Speeding the collaboration between the American Heart Association and the book's publisher, Prentice Hall, were three members of the AHA's Corporate Relations staff: Sam Inman, Debra Ebel, and Ann Yanosky.

AHA Consumer Publications Consultant Peter Landesman assembled the team of experts, writers, and editors. Our managing editor, Jane Ruehl, coordinated the writing, editing, and production. Writer Pat

Naegele transformed the words of the experts into easy-to-read text.

The talented people who created this book were united by a single idea—that people can take control of their health and improve their lives if they have the information they need. Go out and prove them right.

RODMAN D. STARKE, M.D.
Senior Vice President
Office of Scientific Affairs
American Heart Association
National Center

Contents

PART ONE

GENERAL WARRANTY

*What You Need to Know
About You and Your Heart*

PART TWO

SERVICE AND MAINTENANCE
How to Take Care of Your Heart

5   Keep Your Motor Humming with Physical Activity   *129*

PART THREE

HEART CONCERNS
Your Troubleshooting Guide

PART FOUR

GENERAL REPAIRS
What to Do If You Have a Mechanical Breakdown

*I*NTRODUCTION

You know how important it is to take good care of your car. It needs the right fuel, frequent oil changes, and regular maintenance.

In the same way, your body's own engine needs the same care and concern. After all, your heart has to carry you a lot farther for a lot longer. And a heart attack can really stop your engine cold.

As a Heart Owner, you can learn how to keep your body's engine running smoothly for a lifetime. And that's important, because heart disease is America's number one killer, claiming almost a million lives each year.

 ## An Important Message from the American Heart Association

Thanks for selecting this Heart Owner's Manual. It's a one-of-a-kind document. Why? Because it's the first time the American Heart Association has ever explained *everything you need to know* to keep your heart healthy—all in one place.

The information in this Heart Owner's Manual is the result of years of scientific research into what causes heart disease. Literally thousands of studies have shown us the secrets of having a healthy heart. And the good news is: *You can control many of your personal risk factors.*

Years ago, people thought that heart attacks and strokes were things that "just happened," like a lightning bolt from the blue. Today, we know that's not true. We know that your lifestyle habits, to a great extent, determine your risk of developing heart disease. These lifestyle habits are things *you can control.* Things like whether you smoke, what you eat, how much you exercise. how much you weigh, and what your blood pressure is.

The Heart Owner's Manual is easy to use. It's a step-by-step guide on how to keep your heart healthy for life. And following the advice on these pages can make a huge difference in your health and your future.

At the American Heart Association, we're fighting for your life every day. Our mission is to "reduce death and disability from cardiovascular diseases and stroke." This book will help you avoid America's number one killer. It's everything we stand for. Use it in good health.

How to Use This Book

In the pages of this book, you'll learn how your heart works, what helps it, and what hurts it. You'll learn what causes heart attack and stroke—and how to avoid them! You'll also learn the very latest on estrogen replacement and how it fights heart disease, plus new studies on the effects of lowering your blood cholesterol. In short, you'll learn how to make your heart last a lifetime.

 ## Right Off the Showroom Floor

Start by exploring your family's medical history, where you'll learn about your family's history of heart disease. Then find out how your own heart measures up with the Heart Owner's Profile. It will show you if you're living a heart-healthy lifestyle—and what to do to reduce your risk of heart disease.

Finding the Tools You Need

The Heart Owner's Manual guides you step-by-step, with charts and graphs, tests, profiles, and forms designed to help you see where you stand in the race for heart health. Of course, nobody says that changing your lifestyle habits is easy. But, armed with the Heart Owner's Tool Kit, you'll have the tools you need to make all the changes you want.

Healthy Nutrition— The Right Fuel for Your Tank

In the section on "Healthy Nutrition—The Right Fuel for Your Tank" you'll learn how to shop for low-fat, low-cholesterol foods, set up a heart-healthy kitchen, and cook with less fat. You can even eat out at your favorite restaurant and choose foods with your heart in mind—we'll show you how!

Keeping Your Heart Running Smoothly

In the exercise section, we explain how to keep your heart tuned up with regular physical activity. Don't worry, you don't have to run a marathon. We'll show you how to work plenty of activity into your day almost effortlessly. And if you want to exercise, but wonder if it will do any good, check out "The 10 Key Benefits of Physical Activity." It will change your whole point of view! Then we'll start you off with a sample heart-smart walking program.

Customizing Your Chassis

When it comes to losing weight, you'll find out what really works, and why. You'll learn some common fallacies about weight loss, along with the true facts. Plus, we'll give you suggestions on how to build your own personalized weight-loss plan!

How Not to Blow a Gasket

Stress affects us all, and we'll show you how to reduce the negative stresses in your life. And you'll find that improving your communications skills can go a long way toward reducing stress and making your life happier. We'll show you how to relax right down to your toes. Plus we'll look at the common facts and fallacies of emotional health.

Service and Maintenance

Finally, you'll learn about the most common heart and blood vessel problems: what they feel like, how to spot them, and how your doctor can diagnose and treat them. Plus we'll show you just when and how to seek emergency help.

It's all in here—everything you need to know about keeping your heart on the racetrack and out of the pit.

Warnings and Cautions

Look at your car's dashboard. It has gauges and lights to tell you if something is wrong with the engine. The temperature gauge points to "H" if the engine is overheating. A light goes on if the oil pressure is too low. Another gauge shows if your battery is not charging. If you ignore these warning signs, your engine can become so damaged that it stops completely.

The same is true for your own engine, the heart. Certain events and conditions signal that something is wrong—that you might be having a heart attack or stroke. You should know these warning signs so you can take immediate action. The sooner you get help, the less damage you may have.

Warning Signs for Heart Attack and Stroke

Symptoms of a heart attack may vary, but the usual signs are:

- Uncomfortable pressure, fullness, squeezing, or pain in the center of the chest lasting more than a few minutes.
- Pain spreading to the shoulders, neck, or arms; and/or
- Chest discomfort with lightheadedness, fainting, sweating, nausea, or shortness of breath.

You might experience only some of these symptoms. In some cases, the symptoms subside and then return.

Symptoms of a stroke include:

- Sudden weakness or numbness of the face, arm, or leg on one side of the body;
- Sudden dimness or loss of vision, particularly in one eye;
- Loss of speech, or trouble talking or understanding speech;
- Sudden, severe headaches with no apparent cause; and/or
- Unexplained dizziness, unsteadiness, or sudden falls, especially along with any of the previous symptoms.

Action Steps

If you or someone you know experiences any of the symptoms listed above, get medical help right away! Call "911" immediately (if it's available in your area), or contact the fire department or ambulance service. If you can get the person to the hospital quicker by driving yourself, do so. But if you think you are having a heart attack, don't drive. Ask someone to drive you.

The key to survival and recovery is recognizing these signs early and taking action immediately. You'll learn more about the warning signs later in this book. You'll also learn about cardiopulmonary resuscitation (CPR), a mouth-to-mouth breathing and chest compression technique that can keep a heart beating until help arrives.

At the American Heart Association, we hope that you never have to experience "engine failure." That's why we wrote this book. It can help you take care of your heart and reduce your risk of heart attack and stroke. Use it. It can make a difference.

Here's to a long and healthy life!

PART ONE

GENERAL WARRANTY

*What You Need
to Know About You
and Your Heart*

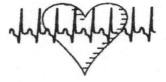

CHAPTER ONE

Building a Healthy Heart Profile

 Looking at Your Model

Automobiles come in all shapes, sizes, and colors, much like people. Different features like engine design, size, manufacturing flaws, fuel injection, or turbo power also distinguish car engines from one another. These features determine how well an engine performs.

Your heart and physiology have unique features that indicate how well your "engine" will perform. These are called heart disease risk factors. These risk factors are linked to an increased risk of developing heart disease. And heart disease greatly diminishes the chance that your heart will perform at an optimal level throughout your lifetime.

The American Heart Association has identified the following major risk factors for heart disease:

- cigarette/tobacco smoking,
- high blood cholesterol,
- high blood pressure,

- physical inactivity,
- heredity,
- male gender, and
- increasing age.

Other contributing factors include diabetes, obesity, and stress.

How to Avoid a Breakdown

Some of these risk factors can be changed to improve your risk of avoiding heart disease. Other factors cannot.

Risk Factors You Can Change

The heart attack risk factors that *can* be changed are cigarette/tobacco smoking, high blood cholesterol, high blood pressure, and physical inactivity. You can also work to avoid obesity and take steps to reduce the stress in your life.

Many of the risk factors are linked with others, so that changing one factor may affect another. For example, increasing your physical activity will reduce your risk. It may also help you lose weight if you burn more calories through activity than you take in through food. This will reduce your risk of heart attack even more! And losing extra weight may help reduce high blood cholesterol and high blood pressure, which will further reduce your heart attack risk.

So, as a Heart Owner, what can *you* do to prevent a heart attack? The first step is to know your risk. The *Heart Owner's Profile* below is designed to help you understand your heart attack risk. The result is simply a "picture" of your overall risk profile. Once you know your risk factors, you can find ways to reduce many of them.

Your Heart Owner's Profile

The Heart Owner's Profile cannot take the place of a complete physical examination by your doctor. Consult your doctor for more thorough evaluation and treatment.

Six key risk factor areas are listed below. Read each one and circle the letter of the statement that is most true for you. After you have completed all six sections, note your answers in the grid on page 10.

	Choose Your Category	**Circle Your Score**
CIGARETTE/TOBACCO SMOKING	Never smoked or stopped smoking three or more years ago	a
	Don't smoke but live or work with smokers	b
	Stopped smoking within last 3 years	c
	Smoke regularly	d
	Smoke regularly and live or work with other smokers	e

Smoking is the single most preventable cause of death. The more you smoke, the higher your risk for heart disease and lung cancer. Your heart disease risk drops dramatically as soon as you quit smoking. About three years after quitting, your risk is almost equal to a person who has never smoked. Quit now. It's never too late. See the section "Clearing the Air—How to Quit Smoking and Start Living," pages 211–229, for information about how to quit smoking.

	Choose Your Category	Circle Your Score
TOTAL BLOOD CHOLESTEROL	Less than 180	a
	180–199	b
Use the number from	Don't know	c
your most recent	200–239	d
blood cholesterol measurement.	240 or higher	e

Too much cholesterol in your blood can clog your arteries and cause a heart attack or stroke. The higher your blood cholesterol level, the higher your risk for clogged arteries. High blood cholesterol can be reduced through changes in diet (see "Healthy Nutrition," pages 57–128), weight loss if you are overweight, and medication if needed. Blood cholesterol levels tend to increase with age, so don't rely on a measure that was taken more than five years ago.

	Choose Your Category	Circle Your Score
HDL CHOLESTEROL	Over 60	a
Use the number from	50–60	b
your most recent	Don't know	c
HDL cholesterol	35–50	d
measurement.	Less than 35	e

HDL cholesterol is a type of cholesterol in your blood. It has been called the "good" cholesterol because high levels of HDL are linked with a lower risk of heart attack. Doctors think it removes excess cholesterol from your arteries. This lowers the risk of the blood vessels becoming clogged and causing a heart attack. You want your HDL cholesterol level to be high. To increase your HDL cholesterol level, be physically active, lose weight (if you're overweight), and stop smoking.

	Choose Your Category	**Circle Your Score**
SYSTOLIC BLOOD PRESSURE	Less than 120	a
	120–139	b
Use the "first" or	Don't know	c
"highest" number	140–160	d
from your most	161 or higher	e
recent blood		
pressure		
measurement.		

Blood pressure is a measure of how hard your heart has to work to circulate blood through your body. The higher your blood pressure, the higher your risk for a stroke or a heart attack. If you are unsure about your blood pressure number, you may be at risk—and not even know it! Get your blood pressure checked at least every two years. If it's high, your doctor may recommend that you:

- lose weight if you are overweight,
- become physically active,
- restrict the amount of sodium in your diet, and
- reduce or quit drinking alcoholic beverages.

Choose the column (1, 2, or 3) that best describes your usual physical activity habits.

YOUR PHYSICAL ACTIVITY QUOTIENT		
1	**2**	**3**
I AM HIGHLY ACTIVE. My job requires very hard physical labor (such as digging, loading/ unloading heavy objects) at least four hours per day. or I do vigorous activities (jogging, cycling, swimming, etc.) at least three times a week for 30–60 minutes or more. or I get at least one hour of moderate activity such as brisk walking at least four days a week.	I AM MODERATELY ACTIVE. My job requires that I walk, lift, carry, or do other moderately hard work for several hours each day (such as day care worker, stock clerk, busboy). or I spend most of my leisure time each week doing moderate activities such as dancing, gardening, walking, yard work, or housework.	I AM INACTIVE. My job requires that I sit at a desk most of the day. and Most of my leisure time is spent in sedentary activities such as watching TV, reading, or other quiet activities and I seldom work up a sweat, and I cannot walk fast without breathing so hard that I have to stop to catch my breath.

If your physical activity habits are most like: *Your score is:*

Column 1   a
Both 1 and 2   b
Column 2   c
Both 2 and 3   d
Column 3   e

People who are inactive are more likely to have heart attacks than people who are active. But you don't have to be a marathon runner to get health benefits from physical activity. In fact, moderate activities, done often, can reduce your risk for heart attack. People who do more vigorous activities have an even lower heart attack risk. Just remember that doing *something* is better than doing *nothing*! See "Keep Your Motor Humming with Physical Activity," pages 129–210, for more information on physical activity.

	"I think I am . . .	
BODY WEIGHT/ BODY SHAPE Which statement best decribes your body weight?	. . . within 10 pounds of my desirable weight."	a
	. . . 10–20 pounds above my desirable weight."	b
	. . . 21–30 pounds above my desirable weight."	c
	. . . 31–50 pounds above my desirable weight."	d
	. . . more than 50 pounds above my desirable weight."	e

Body weight can be an indicator of how much body fat you have. If you weigh more than what is desirable for your height, most of your extra weight is probably excess body fat. People who are extremely physically active may weigh more than desired but most of the excess weight is muscle, not fat. Those who are overweight because of excess body fat are more likely to have high blood pressure, diabetes, and high blood cholesterol. These factors can raise the risk of developing heart disease. A low-fat diet and regular physical activity can help you reduce body fat. The section "How to Get Rid of Your Spare Tire," pages 230–257, offers more information on losing weight.

Body *shape* may be as important as the amount of body fat you have. Recent studies suggest that the location of fat on the body may affect heart attack risk. For example, if a man's waist is bigger than his hips (waist/hip ratio greater than 1.0), his heart attack risk may be significantly higher than the risk of a man whose waist is smaller than his hips. A woman's waist measurement should be no more than 80 percent of her hip measurement (waist/hip ratio greater than 0.8).

Again, losing body fat through regular physical activity and a low-fat diet may help reduce your waist size and therefore your heart attack risk.

Circle your answers for each factor on the grid below.

HEART OWNER'S PROFILE GRID

	Low		Moderate	High	
Cigarette/Tobacco Smoking	a	b	c	d	e
Total Blood Cholesterol	a	b	c	d	e
HDL Cholesterol	a	b	c	d	e
Systolic Blood Pressure	a	b	c	d	e
Physical Activity	a	b	c	d	e
Body Weight/Body Shape	a	b	c	d	e

If Your Answers Are	Your Heart Attack Risk Is
Mostly a's and b's	Low
Mostly c's or some of each	Moderate
Mostly d's and e's	High

Your answer grid is simply a picture of your overall risk profile. A high-risk profile does not mean that you will have a heart attack in the near future. Nor does a low-risk profile mean that you will never have a heart attack. It simply shows which factors you could change to lower your heart attack risk. And that's something worth knowing!

Remember, your risk profile can change. If it is low now, but you become inactive or your blood cholesterol goes up, your risk will increase. If your profile is high, you can reduce it by changing some of your daily habits. The "Service and Maintenance" section, which begins on page 55, will give you practical suggestions and information to help you make healthful changes in your diet, physical activity level, tobacco use, weight, and coping skills.

Also, keep in mind that other factors affect your heart attack risk. These are factors you *cannot* control or change, but it's important that you know what they are.

Risk Factors You Can't Change

Even though you can't do anything to change or improve the following risk factors, you still need to know about them. Understanding these risk factors will give you a more accurate picture of your total risk.

PERSONAL MEDICAL HISTORY. Certain factors in your medical history can affect your heart attack risk. For example:

- Having diabetes increases your risk for a heart attack.
- If you have already had a heart attack, you are more likely to have another one than someone who has never had a heart attack.
- Temporary chest pain that may radiate out to your neck or shoulders could indicate heart disease.
- Pain in the upper legs during exercise may also be a sign of clogged arteries.

- If you have undergone medical procedures such as bypass surgery and angioplasty, you know that you already have heart disease to some extent.

If you have diabetes, your body cannot produce or respond to insulin properly. In that case, your doctor may prescribe changes in your eating habits, ask you to lose weight, and increase your physical activity. He or she may also prescribe drugs, if necessary, to keep the disease in check. However, despite everything that can be done to control diabetes, it is a contributing factor for heart disease that cannot be changed.

Even though you can't control these factors, you can still reduce your heart attack risk by changing the things you *can* control (smoking, activity level, diet, and body weight).

FAMILY MEDICAL HISTORY. Just as we get our eye and hair color from our parents or grandparents, we also inherit tendencies toward certain medical conditions. For example, if one or both of your parents have high blood cholesterol, you may be more prone to having it as well.

Ask your immediate family members about their health status. Find out if any close blood relatives had a heart attack or stroke or died at an age younger than 55 from heart disease. Find out also if any of them had diabetes or were overweight. Use the table below to summarize your findings. Put a check (✓) mark in each category that applies for each relative.

EXPLORING YOUR FAMILY MEDICAL HISTORY

Relation Name	Heart Attack* or Stroke	High Blood Pressure	High Blood Cholesterol	Diabetes	Overweight
Siblings					
1.					
2.					
3.					
4.					
5.					
6.					
Mother					
Mother's Mother					
Mother's Father					
Father					
Father's Mother					
Father's Father					

*Put two check marks (✓✓) in this category if the relative died of heart disease before the age of 55.

RACE. Certain groups in the population have higher rates of heart disease than others. This is because these groups are prone to having one or more of the risk factors listed above. For example:

- African-Americans and Hispanics are more likely to have high blood pressure than the general population.
- American Indians and Hispanics are more likely to develop diabetes.

It's important for you to be aware of your heritage and how it may affect your health risk.

GENDER. Men are more likely to have heart disease than women, and they have heart attacks earlier in life. But the risk for women changes when they go through menopause:

- After menopause, a woman's risk of heart attack begins to rise steadily and almost reaches that of men in about 10 years.
- The number of deaths from cardiovascular disease in men has declined steadily since 1979. The number of deaths from cardiovascular disease in women has increased for many of these same years.
- Women (before and after menopause) who smoke, have diabetes, high blood cholesterol, high blood pressure, and/or a family history of heart disease have a higher risk for heart disease than women who do not have these risk factors. For more information on women and heart disease, see "Unique Features of Different Models," page 15.

AGE. As people get older, their risk of heart attack increases. More than half of all heart attack victims are age 65 or older. But you can adopt more healthful habits at any age to help reduce your heart disease risk.

While you can't do anything to change your age, family, or personal medical history, race, or gender, it's important for you to know which of these risk factors apply to you. Then focus your risk reduction efforts on the things you *can* change! Most of this book is designed to help you find ways to prevent a heart attack or stroke by changing daily habits to reduce your risk.

Unique Features of Different Models

Some cars get great gas mileage, others are gas hogs. Certain models are known for their quiet, comfortable ride while others give up comfort for rugged power. Even within the same product line, there are different models and styles.

Humans come in "different models," too. This book is for all models. But some of the models have special issues related to cardiovascular disease risk. These models include women, children, people over the age of 65, African-Americans, and Hispanics. If you are one of these models, you'll want to read about the unique features of your particular "model." If you are not one of these models, pick up with "Basic Heart Mechanics" on page 21.

WOMEN. Heart disease is not just a man's disease. Heart attack is the number one killer of American women. Of the over 485,000 heart attack deaths that occur each year, a little over 235,000 are women. Also, nearly 87,000 women die each year from stroke. By comparison, about 44,000 women die each year from breast cancer and about 53,000 from lung cancer.

True, men have more heart attacks than women, and they have them earlier in life. After menopause, however, women's risk of heart attack begins to rise steadily, almost reaching that of men in about ten years. If menopause is caused by hysterectomy (surgical removal of the uterus and ovaries), the risk of heart attack rises sharply. If menopause occurs naturally, the risk develops more slowly.

Scientists believe that the female hormone estrogen offers women some protection against heart disease until menopause. That's because estrogen raises HDL cholesterol and lowers LDL cholesterol levels.

Early research indicated a possible link between taking estrogen and the risk of developing endometrial cancer (cancer of the lining of the uterus). For that reason, the newer estrogen replacement therapy (ERT) protocols combined estrogen with progestin, a synthetic form of progesterone (another female hormone). They hoped that this would cancel the risk of endometrial cancer.

The most recent scientific research shows that both estrogen taken alone and estrogen combined with progestin significantly increased HDL levels and lowered LDL levels. The greatest reductions were with estrogen taken alone and estrogen combined with micronized (natural) progesterone. The study also said that estrogen-progestin combination therapy doesn't cause uterine cancer. However, estrogen taken alone greatly increase the risk of pre-cancerous growths in women with a uterus. ERT also does not cause high blood pressure, as previously feared. The latest findings indicate that the estrogen-progestin therapy also decreases fibrinogen, a blood clotting factor that accompanies stroke and heart attack. Scientists are also concerned that while studies indicate that ERT does not cause breast cancer, it might fuel the growth of pre-existing breast tumors. The issue, however, remains unsolved.

The decision to start ERT must be made by you as an individual and your doctor. This decision should be based on your own medical history. If you have a family history of heart disease or if you have many of the risk factors for heart disease, you may be a good candidate for ERT. You may also want this therapy if you suffer menopausal symptoms such as hot flashes, vaginal dryness, or osteoporosis, the disease characterized by crippling bone loss.

On the other hand, if your risk of heart disease is low, but your risk of breast cancer is high, you may want to avoid estrogen replacement therapy. If your doctor prescribes estrogen without progestin, regular checkups are very important. Be sure to have a gynecological check-up before you start estrogen replacement therapy and regularly thereafter for as long as you are taking the estrogen.

What about oral contraceptives? How do they affect your cardiovascular disease risk? Studies done on the early formulations of the Pill showed that they may have increased the risk of heart disease and stroke, especially in women who had high blood pressure and smoked. Studies on the newer, lower-dose formulations of the Pill suggest that the risk is less. Unfortunately, most studies were done on women under age 35. Therefore, not much is known about the effect of low-dose oral contraceptives on the cardiovascular risk of women over age 35.

There is both good news and bad news about the possible links between birth control pills and cancer. On the one hand, using oral contraceptives may help protect you against cancer of the ovaries and the uterus. On the other hand, there is new concern about the use of the Pill and breast cancer.

Your doctor can help you put the latest scientific evidence in the context of your own medical history and need for birth control. You must weigh the safety and effectiveness of other birth control methods as well as the risks of childbirth itself.

One thing we do know for sure, smoking and using oral contraceptives is a deadly combination, increasing your heart attack risk dramatically. If oral contraceptives are the right choice for you, make every effort not to smoke. If you have high blood cholesterol, you may want to try an oral contraceptive that lowers LDL and raises HDL levels. If you are over 35, you may want to use another form of birth control.

If you are under 35, you don't smoke, and you don't have high blood cholesterol or other cardiovascular disease risk factors, a low-dose oral contraceptive may well be okay. Talk with your doctor to evaluate all the risks and benefits of using the Pill.

Much more research must be done on women and cardiovascular disease. In the meantime, lower your risk as much as possible by changing the risk factors you can. These include high blood cholesterol, high blood pressure, cigarette/tobacco use, and being physically inactive. That's good advice regardless of gender.

CHILDREN. Heart attacks and strokes are very rare in children or adolescents. Instead, the cardiovascular diseases most prevalent in children are congenital heart defects, rheumatic heart disease, and Kawasaki disease (see "Trouble Spots," pages 27–29).

Even though heart attack and stroke are rare in children, evidence suggests that the process leading to those conditions begins in childhood. Therefore, it makes sense to start healthful lifestyle training in childhood to promote improved cardiovascular health in adult life. This includes promoting the following:

- regular physical activity,
- a low-fat, low-cholesterol diet after the age of two,
- smoking prevention,
- appropriate weight for height, and
- regular pediatric medical checkups.

The American Heart Association recommends cardiovascular health education and intervention for parents and health care providers according to the following schedule.

Children observe and absorb a lot as they grow up. Many of the life-long beliefs, values, and habits are learned in childhood from parents, other care-givers, siblings, and peers. Set a good example—practice heart-healthy habits yourself.

THE ELDERLY. As you age, your body becomes more subject to conditions or diseases such as high blood pressure, high blood cholesterol, heart attack, and stroke. But you can reduce your risk of cardiovascular disease, even at an advanced age, by doing the following:

- Eat a balanced, nutritious diet.
- Don't smoke.
- Control your blood pressure.
- Be physically active.
- Achieve and maintain your ideal body weight.
- Get regular medical checkups.
- Take your medications as prescribed.

AFRICAN-AMERICANS. In 1990, death rates from cardiovascular diseases were 45 percent higher in black males than white males. For black women, death rates from cardiovascular diseases were 67 percent higher than for white females.

These differences are due to many factors, including the fact that high blood pressure is more common in African-Americans, is more severe, and occurs earlier in life. It is often not treated early or adequately, and it is more likely to result in serious complications. So, if you're African-American, it's critical to find out if you have high blood pressure. Even young people should have regular blood pressure checkups.

In general, the proportion of people who are overweight is higher among African-Americans, especially black women. Being overweight increases the risk for high blood pressure and diabetes, another contributing factor to cardiovascular disease risk.

If you are African-American, it's important for you

to pay close attention to your blood pressure and body weight levels. If you have high blood pressure, you can try to reduce it by:

- losing weight if you are overweight,
- reducing your salt intake,
- cutting down on your alcohol use,
- becoming more physically active,
- quitting smoking, and
- taking any blood pressure medications your doctor prescribes.

To lose weight, reduce your calorie intake slightly and burn more calories by becoming more physically active. Try eating a low-fat, low-cholesterol diet.

HISPANICS. Statistics show that heart disease is the leading cause of death among Hispanics but the rates are lower than for Caucasians. Interestingly enough, Mexican-Americans seem to have a low rate of heart disease even though, as a population, they tend to have high rates of obesity and diabetes. There is very little other data to help guide Hispanics toward reducing heart disease and stroke rates. Researchers are trying to study this group more closely. Until more is known, reducing cardiovascular disease risk by changing your risk factors is still prudent advice.

HIGHLIGHTS

Risks and Rewards

By now, you know the heart disease risk factors for your particular model. Some of your risk factors can probably be changed; others can't. But one thing's for sure: Knowing your risk factors and working to reduce them can reap big rewards . . . in health . . . in happiness . . . in a longer, more productive life.

CHAPTER TWO

Basic Heart Mechanics

 A Look Under the Hood

When you look under your car's hood, what do you see? All cars, no matter what make, model, or year have an engine. That big, solid part has lots of different tubes going into and coming out of it. It's the engine that powers the car. No engine, no go.

You can't get under your "hood" to look at your body's engine. But, as Figure 1 on the next page shows, your heart has a lot of tubes entering and leaving it as well. The main job of the heart is to keep the body's cells alive by pumping oxygen and nutrients to them via the blood. No heart, no go.

General Specifications

The heart is a strong, muscular pump a little larger than a fist. It is only one part of the larger circulatory system that includes the lungs, arteries, arterioles (small arteries), capillaries, venules (small veins), and veins. The heart is continuously working to move blood throughout the circulatory system including the arteries that feed the heart. In fact, it beats over

21

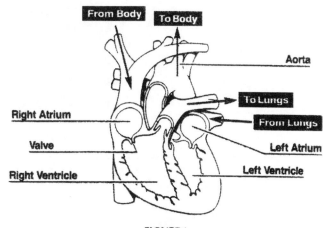

FIGURE 1
The Heart—Your Body's Engine

100,000 times and pumps about 2,000 gallons of blood each day!

Blood from the veins comes into the heart at the right atrium. This is called venous blood. It carries a lot of carbon dioxide but little oxygen. That's because it's returning from the body's tissues where most of the oxygen was removed and carbon dioxide (a waste product) was added. The venous blood goes into the right ventricle and then it is pumped to the lungs. There it gets rid of the carbon dioxide and picks up more oxygen. The oxygenated blood returns to the left atrium and passes into the left ventricle. A strong contraction of the heart muscle sends the oxygenated blood out of the heart, through the aorta, and on its way to nourish the body's tissues. Along the way, waste products are removed as blood is filtered through your kidneys and liver. Figure 2 on the next page shows how extensive your circulatory system is.

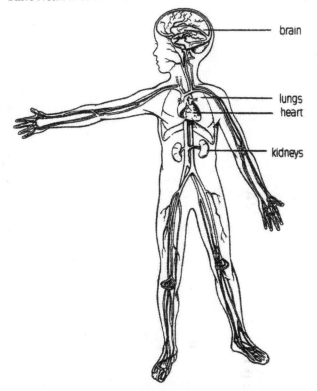

FIGURE 2
Circulatory System

Engine Failure

A number of things can go wrong with your heart and circulatory system in your lifetime. But heart attack and stroke are the most common. A heart attack occurs when the blood supply to part of the heart muscle is severely reduced or stopped (see **Figure 3** on page 24).

This happens when one of the arteries that supplies blood to the heart muscle (called a coronary artery) is blocked or obstructed. Without blood, the heart muscle is not getting oxygen. If the blood supply is cut off drastically or for a long time, the muscle cells "suffocate" and die. (Think of what happens to your car's engine if there is a blockage in the fuel line—it stops cold.) Depending on how much heart muscle is damaged, you may have very little change in your daily function, you may become disabled, or you could even die.

Sometimes a coronary artery temporarily contracts or goes into spasm. When this happens the

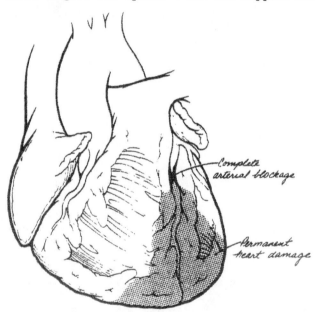

FIGURE 3
Heart with Blockage

artery narrows, and blood flow to part of the heart muscle decreases or even stops. The cause of these spasms is not known, but they can occur in normal coronary arteries as well as ones that are partially blocked.

A stroke occurs when an artery or vein in the brain becomes clogged or bursts. As in a heart attack, a lack of blood to the brain means that oxygen and nutrients are not getting to the brain. In a short period of time, the brain cells die. Recovery from a stroke depends on the amount and location of the damage. Some people recover fully. Others experience some difficulty. Some people find it hard to speak or understand language. Others have memory lapses or paralysis on one side of the body.

Build-Up in the Carburetor

Just like gunk can build up in your car's carburetor, arteries can become blocked, usually as a result of atherosclerosis, a buildup of plaque in the artery walls. Plaque is a substance composed of fatty cholesterol, calcium, fatty substances, and other materials.

Scientists believe that plaque gets started when there is damage to the inside wall of the artery. Possible causes are cigarette smoke, high blood pressure, and high blood cholesterol levels. Once the lining is damaged, fats, cholesterol, and other substances may pass through the damaged lining and become deposited in the artery wall. As these deposits become layered, they begin to narrow the artery, like the buildup of rust inside a pipe. Cells in the artery wall may divide and gradually accumulate, further narrowing the opening of the artery. Figure 4 shows how atherosclerotic plaque can build up over time.

Eventually, this plaque may partially or totally block the blood flow. Or a blood clot can get wedged

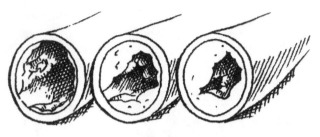

FIGURE 4
Atherosclerotic Plaque

in the narrow opening, completely closing off the vessel. If either of these occurs, there is decreased oxygen to parts of the heart (leading to a heart attack) or brain (leading to a stroke).

 Basic Prevention

As we've discussed, many scientific studies show that certain lifestyle habits actually decrease your risk of coronary heart disease or stroke. These include not smoking cigarettes, maintaining normal blood pressure and blood cholesterol levels, and being physically active. The "Service and Maintenance" section that begins on page 55 offers information and tips on how to change your lifestyle to reduce your risk of heart disease. Other risk factors, such as heredity, gender, medical history (prior heart attack or stroke puts you at greater risk), and increasing age cannot be changed. However, obesity, diabetes, and, possibly, stress are also associated with increased risk for heart disease and stroke. You can help yourself by maintaining your best weight and controlling diabetes. You may also benefit from avoiding situations that are stressful.

The "General Repairs" section, pages 309–346, describes in detail some of the medical procedures required to diagnose and treat a heart attack. Additional information on treating heart attack and stroke is available from your local American Heart Association.

 ## Trouble Spots: Other Types of Heart Disease

Cardiovascular disease is a broad term that incorporates heart diseases and stroke. Heart disease, in turn, is a generalized term for the many disorders affecting the heart. Of these, coronary heart disease or coronary artery disease is the most common type. The American Heart Association's mission is to reduce disability and death due to cardiovascular disease and stroke.

CONGENITAL HEART DEFECTS. A congenital heart defect occurs when the heart or blood vessels near the heart don't develop normally before birth. They are present in almost one percent of live births and are the most frequent congenital malformations in newborns. Obstructions of valves, arteries, or veins and unusual openings between different chambers of the heart are examples of the types of defects that can occur.

In most cases, doctors don't know why they occur. Viral diseases (such as German Measles) or the mother's use of alcohol or drugs during pregnancy are possible causes. Depending on the severity of the defect, doctors may detect it at birth. Other, less severe defects are diagnosed later in infancy. Medication and/or surgery are required to treat heart defects.

RHEUMATIC HEART DISEASE. Rheumatic fever, a result of an untreated strep throat, can permanently damage the heart valves preventing them from opening and closing properly. The damage can vary in severity.

People of any age can develop rheumatic fever, but it usually occurs in children five to fifteen years old. The first symptoms of rheumatic fever are a high fever that lasts ten to fourteen days and arthritic pain that moves from one joint to another. Joints may swell and become hot and red. Children may have shortness of breath or chest pain, indicating that the heart has been affected.

Damage to the heart is not always immediately noticeable. But the damage can eventually become disabling over time. Surgery to replace damaged valves may be necessary.

KAWASAKI DISEASE. This disease tends to strike children (mainly boys and children of Asian ancestry) most often under the age of eight. As many as twenty percent of the children affected with Kawasaki disease have heart damage. Believed to be a virus, Kawasaki disease can weaken the arteries that feed blood to the heart muscle or more rarely cause inflammation of the heart muscle itself. Usually, the disease goes away and permanent coronary artery damage is rare.

CONGESTIVE HEART FAILURE. When the heart is damaged or becomes overworked as a result of high blood pressure, a heart attack, a congenital birth defect, rheumatic fever, or other conditions, blood flow out of the heart slows. The heart simply can't keep blood circulating properly. Blood returning to the heart backs up, causing congestion in the tissues. Kidney function is compromised causing a buildup of sodium and water. Often the legs and ankles swell and fluid may collect in the lungs interfering with normal breathing function.

Congestive heart failure is often treated by medications that reduce fluid retention and allow blood to flow more easily through blood vessels. Dietary restrictions, modified daily activities, and rest are often prescribed as well.

BACTERIAL ENDOCARDITIS. This is a rare, but serious, problem for people who have a heart valve dysfunction or congenital deformation. It is caused by bacteria in the bloodstream that evade the body's normal defenses. They settle on an abnormal or artificial heart valve and can lead to a serious infection of the heart valves or the tissues lining the heart.

Prevention is the best approach. The American Heart Association recommends that people at risk for bacterial endocarditis take antibiotics before:

- undergoing dental procedures that may cause the gums or mouth to bleed,
- having tonsils and adenoids removed, and
- having certain surgeries involving the stomach, intestines, genitals, or urinary tract.

HIGHLIGHTS

Beyond the Basics

Now that you know the basics about this wonderful engine you call your heart, it's time to carry this knowledge a step further. Now, you'll want to know how to keep it operating at peak condition.

CHAPTER THREE

How to Keep Your Heart Finely Tuned

 Your Heart Owner's Tool Kit

Next time you drive your car into a filling station repair bay, look around. You may never have noticed before the huge selection of tools the mechanics have on hand to fix just about any problem that drives through their doors. These include metric wrenches, regular wrenches, diagnostic computers, screwdrivers, pliers, clamps, and other tools and gadgets. All have a specific purpose and often, more than one is needed to fix a problem.

When it comes to changing your behavior to "fix" your cardiovascular disease risk factors, you also have many tools at your disposal.

Shifting Gears

Change. It's a word that can elicit a wide spectrum of feelings. For some people, the process of change is exciting. They like new things: new gadgets for the house, new jobs, new cars. If it's different, they like it.

Other people cringe at the thought of making changes. They like knowing what to expect. Routine feels comfortable to them.

Reducing the risk of heart disease and stroke may involve changing one or more of your daily habits. The "Heart Owner's Profile" assessment, page 10, showed you the specific areas that you could change. If you're comfortable with change, you might feel like jumping in right away with these risk reduction changes.

> "Good-bye couch potato! From now on, I'm going to exercise every day!"
> "Fried foods and rich desserts are forever banished from my plate."
> "I am finally going to become a nonsmoker."

Sounds a lot like a New Year's resolution list, doesn't it? And we all know what happens to resolutions by the end of January.

On the other hand, you may not be comfortable with change. Or you think changing some of your daily habits is going to be too difficult. These perceptions could keep you from taking the first step toward realizing the health benefits of risk reduction strategies.

That's why it is important to understand the process of change. New research is suggesting that there is one reason people have not been successful in initiating or maintaining healthful behavior changes. It is because they force themselves to change before they are truly ready.

Researchers have studied people who have been successful at making lifestyle changes such as quitting smoking. How and why did these people attain their goals? What researchers learned is that, in order to be successful, people need to progress through a series of steps or stages in the change process. We're calling these necessary stages neutral, first gear, second gear, third gear, fourth gear, and high gear. Like driving a standard transmission car, each gear is dependent on the one before. If you turn on the engine, put your foot on the clutch, and immediately shift into high gear, what happens? You stall out! To get to high gear successfully, you have to start out in first, gradually pick up speed, then shift to second. After picking up a little more speed, you shift to third, to fourth, and finally to high gear. Soon you are cruising down the highway, not having to worry any longer about shifting.

The same seems to be true for people making changes. If you want to make a change, you have to start out in first gear, the earliest stage. Then gradually move through the other gears until you reach a "cruising speed." That is where the change has become a permanent part of your life. This gearing up for change can be applied to any behavior change: becoming more active, reducing fat in your diet, or quitting smoking.

How ready for change are you? The stages in the change process are described below.

Neutral Gear

Have you ever thought about making a change? If not, you're in neutral gear. Scientists call this the precontemplation stage. You may be unaware of the need to change or, if you are aware, you feel that the "cons" of changing outweigh the "pros" of changing. For example, you may feel that the benefit you might gain from walking 30 minutes each day is not worth the time it takes away from your work and family.

Often, people in neutral are defensive about changing. They may be demoralized by previous attempts to change. They may not see the value in changing or are simply not interested in changing. To force people who are in neutral to do something that is action-oriented (like starting to exercise) is like switching into fourth gear from a dead stop—they're going to stall out.

First Gear

The next gear is when you are seriously thinking about taking some action in the near future. "I need to start watching my diet since my cholesterol level is high" or "I really want to lose some weight" are statements typical of a person in first gear. Scientists call this the contemplation stage. In this gear, there is some interest, but still there are doubts and disadvantages that keep the person from acting on these desires. People can get stuck in this stage for a long time, even years. We all know someone who keeps saying, "Someday I am going to _____." (You can insert just about any behavior in the blank.) Yet, time flies by and they fail to make any attempt to change.

Second Gear

If you've been in first gear and you've tried the new behavior at least once in the last year, you've slipped into second gear. Scientists call this the preparation stage. A person who starts an exercise program for two weeks, then stops for two months, then starts up again for three weeks is in second gear. People in this gear make a conscious choice to change the problem behavior. For example, they may seek help from a doctor, join a group, or develop their own strategies for change. They just can't sustain the effort for very long.

Third Gear

This is the gear in which the person is consistently practicing the new behavior. Scientists call it the action stage, and it lasts at least six months. Researchers found that, in general, most people do stay in third gear long enough. If a person loses his or her vigilance before the end of the six-month period, they are likely to relapse into their old behavior. Third gear is where many of the habit-changing tools described in the next section will come in handy.

Fourth Gear

When a person has maintained the new behavior for about six months, they then move into fourth gear, which scientists call the maintenance stage. Fourth gear lasts until you're in high gear, and it can vary a great deal in length. In fourth gear, the person continues to practice the new behavior. They may have occasional lapses, but these occur less often as time goes on. People in fourth gear are able to quickly bounce back from a relapse.

High Gear

While many people may eventually reach fourth gear, relatively few truly shift into high gear. In high gear, which scientists call the termination stage, a person does not feel any temptation to relapse into the old behavior. Also, the person has absolute confidence that he or she will not revert to the old behavior, regardless of the situations that may arise. For example, an ex-smoker feels totally confidant that he or she will not smoke again. Or a regularly active person would not be tempted to be sedentary during an extended vacation. In high gear, you've arrived. You don't have to worry about shifting to another gear.

Remember that people are at different places when it comes to making lifestyle changes. It is entirely possible that you could be in different gears for changing each heart disease risk factor you want to alter. For example, you could be in third gear (the action stage) when it comes to low-fat eating but still be in second gear (the contemplative stage) when considering an increase in physical activity. Also, it's normal for people to "shift back" or relapse to an earlier stage.

When you recognize what gear you're in, you can work to shift to the next gear. Remember, you'll improve your chances of success if you shift gears sequentially and if you allow yourself time to experience each gear fully.

Use the following "Gearing Up For Change Profile" to help you decide where you are in relation to each behavior. Pick the number that best describes the way you currently feel.

Gearing Up for Change Profile

A. Smoking

1. I am currently smoking, and I do not intend to quit in the next six months.
2. I am currently smoking, but I intend to quit in the next six months.
3. I am currently smoking, but I intend to quit in the next month.
4. I have not smoked for the past six months.
5. I quit smoking more than six months ago.
6. I have never smoked and I am confident that I never will.

B. *Heart-Healthy Diet**

1. I am not eating a heart-healthy diet, and I do not intend to adopt one in the next six months.
2. I am not eating a heart-healthy diet, but I do intend to adopt one in the next six months.
3. I am not eating a heart-healthy diet, but I do intend to adopt one in the next month.
4. I have been eating a heart-healthy diet for less than six months.
5. I have been eating a heart-healthy diet for more than six months.
6. I have been eating a heart-healthy diet for more than six months and I am confident that I will continue this diet no matter what roadblocks come up.

C. *Physical Activity*

1. I am not physically active, and I do not intend to become active in the next six months.
2. I am not physically active, but I intend to become more active in the next six months.
3. I am not physically active, but I intend to become more active in the next month.
4. I have been physically active for less than the past six months.
5. I have been physically active for more than the last six months.
6. I have been physically active for more than 6 months and I am confident that I can continue no matter what roadblocks come up.

---

*In this diet, less than 30 percent of daily calories are from fat and less than 10 percent of daily calories are from saturated fat. It also contains no more than 300 milligrams of cholesterol per day and no more than 3,000 milligrams of soldium per day.

Find the number you circled for each of the behaviors listed above. Using the following key, rank your stage of change for each of the areas described above:

1 = Neutral Gear
2 = First Gear
3 = Second Gear
4 = Third Gear
5 = Fourth Gear
6 = High Gear
7 = Does not apply to me
A. Smoking   _____
B. Heart-Healthy Diet   _____
C. Physical Activity   _____

Heart disease risk factors such as high blood cholesterol and high blood pressure are not included in the "Gearing Up for Change Profile" because they are conditions, not behaviors. However, changing the behaviors listed above can positively impact blood cholesterol, blood pressure, body weight, and diabetes.

It works best to choose one area to work on at a time. Start with a behavior in which the profile shows you are in the preparation or action stage. Depending on the behavior you target for change, you may want to use more than one of the tools listed below. And you may find that some of these tools are more useful at different times than others.

 ## Tracking Your Lifestyle Habits

Research shows that people who are aware of their daily habits and who keep track of their progress are more likely to succeed in changing health behaviors than those who do not. Self-monitoring is a simple process in which you write down your activities and behaviors for a specific period of time.

Short-Term Maintenance

In the beginning, tracking your behavior can be very helpful in identifying and understanding your habits. For example, you may think that you are eating a low-fat diet. But after tracking your eating habits and calculating your fat intake for several days, you may find you are eating much more fat than you thought. Or after tracking your physical activity for several weeks, you may come to realize that you aren't as sedentary as you thought. Even if you don't "work out" on a regular basis, you may be getting a fair amount of moderate-level physical activity. You can do that just by working in your garden and walking your dog twice a day.

John had been a smoker for 23 years. He had attempted to quit on his own countless times, mostly by trying to go "cold turkey." But he could never go more than a week without lighting up again.

John decided to enroll in a smoking cessation class to learn other tactics that might help him quit. One of the first things he learned was how to track his smoking habits. To do this, he wrapped a piece of paper around his pack of cigarettes and held it in place with a rubber band. Every time he reached for a cigarette, he wrote down the time, location, what he was doing, and what he was feeling before and after he smoked.

After doing this for several days, John could identify several patterns to his smoking. The tracking sheet showed that he tended to smoke when he was tense or bored. Smoking seemed also to be tied to talking on the phone. Having identified these triggers, John learned several relaxation techniques and created a list of fun things he can do when he gets bored. Since talking on the phone is essential to his job, John had to substitute a new behavior for smoking. Now when the phone rings, he grabs a soft rubber ball and squeezes it throughout the conversation. •

Forms for tracking eating, physical activity, and smoking behaviors are provided in Appendix B. Make photocopies of these forms and use them to help identify your current habits and track changes that you make over time.

Long-Term Maintenance

At times, changing your behavior can seem like a slow process. You'll experience plateaus and lapses that make you feel like you're getting nowhere. But keeping track of your status over time can help remind you of the progress you have made. After all, nothing motivates like success!

Eight years ago, Cathy discovered that her total blood cholesterol level was 223 mg/dl. The doctor told Cathy to reduce her saturated fat and cholesterol intake, to lose weight, and to work more physical activity into her daily lifestyle. Cathy implemented some changes. Six months later she returned to her doctor for a follow-up visit. Her cholesterol level had dropped to 198 mg/dl, which pleased both Cathy and her doctor.

Every year since then, Cathy has had her cholesterol checked. She has tracked the results on a graph similar to the one shown in Appendix B. Tracking her cholesterol level over time has helped her recognize her success. It also shows her that when she slacks off on her diet or activity level, her cholesterol level tends to rise a little. When that happens, she knows she has to be a little more vigilant with her daily habits. ●

Graphs for tracking changes in blood cholesterol, blood pressure, and weight status over the long term are included in Appendix A. Think of these forms as "Maintenance Logs" similar to the ones you use to keep track of the different services performed on your car. A recommended "Maintenance Schedule" for each area is provided in the beginning of Appendix A

 Managing Triggers

Often what you do or think is preceded by an event or feeling. Most of the time, you are not even aware of your "triggers." That's why tracking your behavior for several days or a week is important. Self-monitoring can help you identify specific triggers that cause certain behaviors.

Triggers may arise when you are with certain people or in social situations such as parties or meetings. For example, you may smoke more when you are at a happy hour with your friends. These are called "social" cues. Other things in your environment may trigger your behaviors, too. "External" cues can include, but are not limited to the following:

- the smell or sight of certain foods;
- watching TV (What do you usually do when a commercial comes on?);
- a certain place (When was the last time you skipped the popcorn at the movie theater?); and
- a certain time (How often do you have a "bed time snack" even though you are not really hungry?).

You may also experience "internal" cues that can trigger unhealthful behaviors. These internal cues include the way you feel and the way you talk to yourself. What happens when you're feeling anxious, lonely, or depressed? How do you respond after you have told yourself, "I am too tired to exercise" or "I don't have time to be active"? Do any of these trigger you to smoke, drink alcohol, overeat, or skip your exercise?

Mary has been working hard to lose weight. However, someone in the family has left a box of her favorite cookies on the counter. The sight of the cookies triggers her desire to eat some. After her seventh cookie, Mary is feeling guilty for "blowing her diet." Her guilt turns into self-loathing because she feels she has no willpower. The negative feelings eat at her self-confidence and soon she labels herself a failure. The negative self-talk triggers Mary to continue eating until she finally finishes off the rest of the cookies.

Once you know your triggers you can develop strategies to either avoid the triggering situations or find ways to adapt to them. For example, Mary could have eliminated her trigger by asking her family to keep "high-risk" foods out of her sight.

June gets really nervous when she goes to her in-laws' home for the holidays. The nervousness causes her to overeat. To deal with this trigger she can refuse to go (not a realistic option) or she can develop some strategies to cope with her nervousness. June decides that she will practice deep breathing to reduce stress at least three times each day while she is at her in-laws. She also promises herself that she will go for a walk when she gets really nervous and is at risk of pigging out. ●

George had a ritual each Monday and Friday morning. He would stop at the doughnut shop on his way to work. George liked the attention and words of appreciation he received from his colleagues when he brought doughnuts. Unfortunately, having the doughnuts around the office was a trigger for him (and others) to eat.

George completely eliminated this trigger by taking a different route to work. That way, he wasn't tempted to stop by his regular doughnut shop. After several weeks, he realized that he missed the attention he received when he brought doughnuts to the office. He was about to return to his habit of bringing doughnuts again. Then it occurred to him that his co-workers would probably appreciate healthful snacks as much as they did the doughnuts.

So George started to bring in low-fat muffins and fruit on Mondays and Fridays. Sure enough, his colleagues loved the new, healthful treats. Having food around is still a trigger to eat. At least now George and his friends munch on low-fat, low-cholesterol goodies instead of high-fat sweets. ●

One person's trigger may not be a problem for someone else. That's why it's important for you to know what your triggers are. Review your dietary, physical activity, and smoking logs to identify and understand your triggers.

WHAT SETS YOUR TRIGGERS OFF?

Trigger	Avoid?		Strategies for Changing My Response to This Trigger
	Yes	No	

Also, you can use other triggers to help you adopt and maintain healthful behaviors. For example, you can keep a pair of comfortable shoes sitting out near your door at work to remind you to be active during the workday. Or you might try putting a fruit bowl on the counter or keeping cut-up vegetables in a clear container in the refrigerator. These triggers may prompt you to include more of these foods in your diet.

Recruiting Support— A Gold Mine of Positive Reinforcement

Friends, family, coworkers, neighbors, social groups, clubs, teachers, support groups, etc. can help you reach your heart disease and stroke risk reduction goals. They can simply offer you words of encouragement, or they may be willing to participate in your new habits. For example, a neighbor may be willing to walk with you each day, or a family member may be willing to join you in eating low-fat meals.

Teachers, mentors, counselors, and coaches can help you gather information and acquire skills that will help support and sustain your new habits. But sometimes all you need is someone to listen non-judgmentally to your concerns and problems.

In order to get the help you need, you must ask for it. This is difficult for a lot of people because they think that asking for assistance is a sign of weakness. Or it may sound as if they're imposing. If you have difficulty asking people to help you, think about the times when you gave a helping hand to a friend. How did it make you feel to know that you made a difference in that person's life? Chances are, you felt pretty good.

Sometimes people don't know how to ask for help. There are two keys to getting support. One is to identify what you feel will help you attain your goals. The other is to identify who is the best person or group to help you. When you actually ask for their help, be very specific about how they can help you. Afterwards, remember to show your appreciation. No, you don't have to give each of them a sports car. A simple, heartfelt "Thank you, I really appreciate your help" is more than enough. Use the chart on the next page to plan out your strategies for recruiting help and support.

REACHING OUT FOR HELP			
Problem/Issue I Need Help With	Person(s) Who Could Help	How He/She Could Help	How I Can Thank Him/Her

Sally's doctor prescribed a low-fat, low-cholesterol diet to help lower her blood cholesterol level. Her family agreed to try lower-fat menus to help support her efforts. After about six months, Sally had her cholesterol level under control and was enjoying an added bonus of a slight weight loss.

Her husband, Kyle, was supportive of his wife's efforts at first. But after she had lost twenty pounds, he began to worry that she would become more attractive to other men and that she would leave him. He became preoccupied with this irrational fear and subconsciously began to sabotage Sally's maintenance efforts. He started bringing home her favorite ice cream, leaving potato chip bags on the counter, and insisting on eating out at places that had limited menus. Until Sally confronted him with how his actions were affecting her, he didn't realize what he was doing. When she asked Kyle to reinforce his pledge of support, Sally learned of his concerns about her leaving him. A few sessions of marriage counseling and more open communication helped Sally and Kyle work things out. ●

Setting Goals:
4 Steps to a Healthier You

It may sound overly simplistic to emphasize the need to set goals, but it is surprising how few people actually do it. And those who try to set goals often do an incomplete job. There are many different goal-setting models to choose from. Find one that works for you. Goal-setting strategies can help you do the following: determine where you want to be, see where you are, reach your goal, and review your plans.

Determining Where You Want to Be

Much too often, people set a goal and expect that, somehow, it will just happen. There's more to goal setting than that. First, is your goal realistic? Don't expect that you can go from being totally sedentary to running a marathon in three months. Consider your history, the resources you have, and your stage of readiness to change.

Next, make sure the goal is yours. If you are doing something because someone else wants you to—even if it's your doctor—you will not be as committed to it as if it was wholly your goal. Closely examine the pros and cons of attaining the goal. If your cons outweigh someone else's pros, you are still in neutral gear (see page 32) and not likely to be successful.

Third, be sure the goal is measurable. If you say your goal is to, "lower my blood pressure" how will you know when you have reached it? A one millimeter of mercury reduction would qualify, but is that enough to make a difference in your health? A better goal statement would be, "At my next doctor's visit in six months (cite a date), I will have lowered my blood pressure to less than or equal to 132 over 82."

Seeing Where You Are

It's important to assess your current status relative to your goal. This way you'll know how much of a gap there is between where you are now and your eventual goal. Knowledge of the gap then drives the next step in goal-setting. Refer to your Heart Owner's Profile results for information about your current status.

Reaching Your Goal

It is sometimes easier to start at the final goal and work backwards step-by-step to your current state. Again, be realistic with your plans and mini-goals. You want to challenge yourself, but not so stringently that you set yourself up to fail.

Reviewing Your Goals and Plans

If you keep your goals in your head, chances are you will forget them or subconsciously change them over time. Write them down where you can easily access them. Some people post their goals and plans on the bathroom mirror. Others keep them in their wallet, purse, or calendar. Set specific dates and times for reviewing your progress. Remember, it's okay to slightly modify your plans if it will help you attain your goal.

Rewarding Yourself: Acknowledging Your Worth

A common mindset of people attempting health promotion goals is, "I don't need to reward myself. I should quit smoking because it is good for me. That should be reward enough." If such thinking is true, why haven't more people adopted healthful behaviors? The truth is, rewards are important.

Finding a way to reward yourself is a way of saying to yourself, "Hey, I'm important. I matter." It's hard for some people to affirm themselves like this, but it's important to regularly reward your progress.

A reward can be anything that is particularly motivating to you. You may save for a trip by putting a dollar in a jar on your dresser every day after you have completed at least 15 minutes of physical activity. Maybe you would like to treat yourself to a facial for eating at least five fruits and vegetables almost every day for a week.

A couple of precautionary words about rewards. Identify your reward at the time you set your goal. If you are trying to lose weight or lower your blood cholesterol level, don't use high-fat foods as your reward. You may trigger a relapse or, if nothing else, take in a lot of empty calories. Instead, include these foods in your usual diet *in moderation* and reward yourself with a non-food treat.

Make sure your rewards are commensurate with the goal or mini-goal that you attain. Staying smoke-free for one year is more deserving of a scuba-diving trip to Mexico than achieving your physical activity goals for three days. But a 30-minute, undisturbed soak in the tub would be perfect for the latter. Appendix A contains a sample behavior change contract you can use for setting any behavior change goals.

In the spaces provided below, brainstorm all the different rewards you could give yourself for attaining your health-related goals. Think big and small, extravagant and simple. Photocopy the list and post it where you will regularly see it. Some of the things you list here may be just what you need to motivate you to change something you have been intending to change for a long time.

MY REWARD LIST

1.	21.
2.	22.
3.	23.
4.	24.
5.	25.
6.	26.
7.	27.
8.	28.
9.	29.
10.	30.
11.	31.
12.	32.
13.	33.
14.	34.
15.	35.
16.	36.
17.	37.
18.	38.
19.	39.
20.	40.

Thinking Positively— A Key to Self-Esteem

We talk to ourselves constantly. No, usually not out loud. Quietly, inside our own heads. Most of the time we're not even aware of what we are saying. But a lot of what we tell ourselves shows up in the way we act and what we feel.

Self-talk is a powerful reinforcer of self-esteem. For example, the record inside your head may be constantly telling you that you don't have time to be physically active. If that's the case, then you won't have time. You won't even try to find the time to be active. Or perhaps you have convinced yourself that if you can't do at least 45 minutes of physical activity every day, then you might as well do nothing at all. Such all-or-none thinking is a common self-talk trap. But rarely are things in life so black and white.

Another example of negative self-talk is when you lapse slightly. Maybe you had half a box of cookies in one sitting. People with low self-esteem will tend to magnify the significance of such an event. A magnified response to over-eating cookies might be, "Oh no, I have really blown it! I've just ruined all my hard work for the last six months!" In reality, how likely is it that the calories contained in one-half of a box of cookies are going to wipe out all the positive changes made to date? Not likely. Magnifying (or minimizing) events is an example of irrational thinking that often generates negative self-talk.

The flip side of self-talk contains positive thoughts and affirmations that boost self-esteem. Back to the cookie example, here's a positive and more rational response. "Wow. I ate more than I planned. I am disappointed, but I know lapses like this will happen from time to time. I've made great progress to this point. I'll be more careful for the next couple of days."

The first step in combating negative self-talk and boosting self-esteem is to become aware of your conversations with yourself. Think about what you say to yourself before, during, and after a challenging time. You may already be aware of some of your broken-record statements. If not, try recording your thoughts for one or two weeks. You might be surprised at what you hear.

As you become more aware, start to catch your negative thoughts before they fully develop. Then ask yourself if the thought is accurate and true. Try turning it around to be more rational and positive. The goal is not to keep you from talking to yourself. It is to make the conversations more rational, supportive, and positively affirming.

Preventing Relapse

Changing life-long habits is rarely a "cold turkey" proposition. Remember the "Shifting Gears" concept (see pages 30–37)? In fact, it is very much a "two steps forward, one step backward" process. That means we can expect to experience roadblocks or challenges that cause us to stray from our plans and goals. The key, however, is to keep such lapses very short-term and to find ways to get back on track quickly. Otherwise, one lapse can lead to another. Successive lapses become a relapse. A prolonged relapse can lead to a collapse—total return to the original behavior.

Recognizing High-Risk Situations

As discussed in a previous section, there are situations, people, and places that are particularly troublesome for each of us. Not everyone has difficulty with the same high-risk situations. That's why it's important to know what things set you back and trigger undesirable behaviors. Once you are aware of these situations, you can plan strategies for coping with them.

Maria was feeling really good about her new walking program. For the past three weeks, she walked for 30 minutes each weekday. One morning, it was pouring rain, and Maria was nearly in a panic because she couldn't get outside to walk. She began to think that she had "failed" because she missed her walk. All day long she carried a heavy burden of guilt and disappointment.

When she got home that night, she calmed down and looked rationally at the situation. She knew that her part of the country was about to start its "rainy" season, so the morning's experience was going to happen again. To prepare herself for the "high-risk" event caused by rain, Maria made some contingency plans:

- Drive to a mall and walk inside for 30 minutes.
- Buy a rain poncho and dig out an older pair of sneakers so that she can go walking and enjoy the rain.
- Allow herself to skip one session a month due to rain. ●

Practicing Effective Coping Strategies

Even with "high-risk" contingency plans in place, lapses are still going to occur from time to time. The key is to limit the severity and duration of a lapse by practicing effective coping strategies. These include many of the behavioral skills discussed previously. Self-tracking can help you:

- see what caused you to falter,
- recruit help,
- review and reaffirm your goals and plans,
- think positively, and
- remind yourself of your rewards.

Other strategies are to outlast urges and remove yourself from the situation, if possible. Urges to eat, smoke, or be inactive occur all the time, especially in the beginning of your behavior change efforts. If you examine urges closely, they all look similar. That is, they are composed of the same parts. At first there is a little twinge or awareness that you want to smoke, overeat, or skip being active. Gradually, the urge builds in intensity, consuming more of your thoughts and attention as time goes on. But it's important to know that the intensity of the urge will almost always subside if you can outwait it. Try to distract yourself when you feel an urge coming on.

Dominick is trying to be active at least five days a week. He found that the best time to fit activity into his schedule is right after he gets home from work. Often, when he is driving home, he feels the urge to scrap his exercise plans and just plop down in front of the TV until dinner.

He has become aware of this problem, so now as soon as he starts to feel this urge, he changes the car radio to a rock and roll station and turns it up loud. When he gets home, he immediately changes into his exercise shorts and shoes without even thinking about whether or not he wants to exercise. Usually, by the time he has finished lacing up his shoes, the urge to be inactive has passed and he heads out the door. ●

Sometimes the only way to stifle a lapse is to remove yourself from the situation.

Sam was a recent ex-smoker who joined his buddies at a happy hour after work. As he entered the bar, Sam smelled cigarette smoke. He never realized how smoke-filled and tempting bars and clubs are. As he made his way to the table where his friends were sitting, he became aware of the urge to bum a cigarette and light up. Sam was not confident that he could wait out the urge, so he made up an excuse and left the bar immediately. ●

It's not always possible to remove yourself from the troublesome situation. But keep it in your behavior change tool kit for those occasions when it is appropriate.

HIGHLIGHTS ─────────────────────────────

Tools for Change

Now you have the tools you need to help you decide on a goal, get support, and keep yourself on track until the new behavior becomes second nature. In the next chapter we'll talk about one of the most targeted areas for change: diet and nutrition.

PART TWO

SERVICE AND MAINTENANCE

*How to Take Care
of Your Heart*

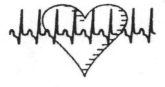

CHAPTER FOUR

Healthy Nutrition—
The Right Fuel
for Your Tank

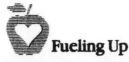 Fueling Up

A car's engine needs the right kind of gasoline to make the pistons move, which turns the drive train, which, in turn, makes the wheels move. In the same way, your heart needs the right kind of fuel so it can accomplish its very important task. That is to pump the blood that carries nutrients and oxygen to every part of your body.

Fuel for your heart and other body tissues comes from the foods you eat. And eating a healthful diet is important. Nutritious foods give your body the nutrients and energy it needs to do the following:

- maintain and repair tissues,
- keep the basic body processes (breathing, digesting, and pumping blood) functioning, and
- work and play every day.

Healthful, low-fat foods keep your engine stoked with fuel for the long haul. There are six classes of nutrients: carbohydrate, protein, fat, vitamins, minerals, and water. The first three provide calories, a way of fueling the body's energy supply. Alcohol also provides calories, but it is not considered a nutrient because it provides "empty" calories, much the same as sugar. The different calorie sources supply different amounts of energy:

- Fat   9 Calories per gram
- Alcohol   7 Calories per gram
- Carbohydrate   4 Calories per gram
- Protein   4 Calories per gram

When a food label shows that one serving contains 100 calories, that means it contains protein, fat, carbohydrate, or alcohol in some combination that adds up to 100 calories. Vitamins and minerals do not supply energy but they are nonetheless very important in maintaining good health. Vitamins are necessary for normal metabolism, but the body cannot make them in adequate amounts. A deficiency in any one of them can lead to disease symptoms. Fortunately this can be corrected by adding that vitamin to your diet.

 AHA Fueling Recommendations

Research over the past few decades has shown scientists the role that diet plays in the treatment and prevention of coronary heart disease. Based on this research, the American Heart Association recommends that adults eat foods that are low in fat, especially saturated fat, and cholesterol.

Why? Because these nutrients tend to increase the amount of cholesterol in the blood. And cholesterol from the blood can line the innermost layer of an artery that has been damaged. This is the beginning of a disease called atherosclerosis, which can eventually stop the flow of blood. When this happens in an artery leading to the heart, that's a heart attack. When it happens in an artery leading to the brain, that's called a stroke.

The AHA also recommends that most people take it easy on salt (sodium). In some people, too much sodium in the diet may contribute to high blood pressure, another major risk factor for heart disease.

The American Heart Association has adopted the following dietary guidelines for all healthy people two years old and older.

- Keep your total fat intake to less than 30 percent of daily calories.
- Limit saturated fat to less than 10 percent of total calories.
- Limit polyunsaturated fat to no more than 10 percent of calories.
- Use monounsaturated fat to make up the rest of total fat intake (about 10 to 15 percent of calories).
- Limit your cholesterol intake to no more than 300 milligrams per day.
- Keep sodium intake to no more than 3000 milligrams (3 grams) per day.
- If you drink alcohol, limit yourself to fewer than two drinks per day.
- Maintain a healthful body weight.
- Eat a wide variety of foods.

When Josie went in for her yearly physical, she was told that her blood pressure and cholesterol levels were higher than they were the previous year. The doctor told her to reduce her fat intake to between 20 and 30 percent of calories. He emphasized cutting saturated fat and cholesterol levels as well. As Josie was about to ask some questions about diet, her doctor hurriedly turned and walked out the door. He said over his shoulder, "I'll see you in a year."

Dazed and confused, Josie had no idea what "30 percent of calories" meant in terms of food choices. So she contacted her local American Heart Association office and asked for information. Josie now knows how to eat a better diet. ●

People eat food, not numbers. So how do you know if you are actually eating a heart-healthy diet?

 ## Evaluating Your Eating Habits

The chart below gives you a chance to check up on your eating habits. It describes three very different eating patterns, each broken down into food groups. In each food group, circle the list of foods (column A, B, or C) that most closely matches how you usually eat. You may choose two lists, if applicable. This will give you a profile of your current eating habits.

 YOUR EATING PATTERNS AT A GLANCE
(Choose One)

Food Groups	A	B	C
Bread, Cereals and Other Starchy Foods	Whole-grain breads, bagels, most cereals, rice, pasta, corn tortillas, beans prepared without added fat	Cornbread, muffins, regular crackers, egg noodles, flour tortillas, beans prepared with fat	Doughnuts, biscuits, croissants, pastries, high-fat crackers

Food Groups	A	B	C
Fruits and Vegetables	5 or more servings* per day	2-4 servings* per day	Less than 2 servings* per day
Dairy Products	Nonfat or skim milk, yogurt, and cheese	Low-fat (1-2% milk fat) milk, yogurt, and cheese	Whole milk, whole-milk yogurt and cheese
Meats, Poultry, Fish, Eggs	Small portions of lean beef and pork cuts; poultry without skin; seafood, fish; egg whites	Large portions of lean beef and pork cuts, poultry with skin, lean lunch meats, whole eggs	Marbled beef and pork, bacon, sausage, bologna, hot dogs, fried chicken and fried fish, canned fish-packed in oil
Fats and Oils	I rarely add fats and oils when preparing foods at home.	I often add fats and oils when preparing foods at home.	I always add fats and oils when preparing foods at home.
Desserts and Snacks	Pretzels, angel food cake, graham crackers, fig bars, low-fat crackers and cookies, low-fat popcorn, non-fat frozen yogurt	Low-fat chips, cakes, brownies, regular popcorn, ice milk, or sherbet	Regular potato, corn, and cheese chips; rich cakes, cookies and pies; ice cream

* One serving = 1 medium piece of fruit, 1/2 cup chopped or cooked fruit or vegetables, 3/4 cup fruit or vegetable juice, 1 cup raw leafy greens

TEST RESULTS. Now look to see which column (A, B, or C) most of your circled food lists fall into.
   If your eating habits are most like:

Column A | Congratulations! You are enjoying a low-fat diet that may help reduce some of your risk factors for heart attack and stroke. Keep up the good work!

Both A and B | You are doing a pretty good job of keeping the fat in your diet low, but you could do better! Make a few more changes so that more of your food choices are from Column A.

Column B | Your diet is moderately high in fat. You may have made some steps in the right direction. Keep making changes slowly so that most of your food choices are from Column A.

Both B and C | Your diet is probably higher in fat than is healthy for you. Try to move away from some foods in the Column C pattern, and eat them only once in a while. Make changes slowly so that more of your choices are from Column B, then mostly from Column A.

Column C | Your diet is much too high in fat! This may increase some of your risk factors for heart disease. Choose one or two food groups and start slowly to make changes toward Column B, then Column A. Save the Column C foods to eat only once in a while.

So now you know how your diet stacks up against what the American Heart Association recommends. But are you ready to make some changes in your diet? Refer back to the "Heart-Healthy Diet" section of the "Gearing Up for Change Profile" quiz on page 35. If you are in neutral gear, examine why you haven't really thought about changing your diet. Do you think it is not important? If so, review the section, "American Heart Association Fueling Recommendations," on pages 58–59. Do you think it is too much trouble? The ideas in this chapter may surprise you by how practical and simple they are.

If you are in first gear, think about why you have not taken any steps to improve your diet. Is it because you don't have the tools or the information about how to work heart-healthy habits into your daily routine? If so, read on. This chapter is full of practical ideas for making heart-healthy eating easy and delicious.

If you are in second or third gear, congratulations on trying to improve your diet. You may already be doing some of the things that are recommended in this chapter. Still, there may be techniques and suggestions that will improve your heart-healthy eating efforts even more. If you are in fourth gear, you may also benefit from reviewing basic heart-healthy eating strategies.

Some people say, "You are what you eat." There's a bit of truth to that. The foods you eat do not directly affect your risk of heart disease or stroke. But they may affect your blood cholesterol, blood pressure, and body fat levels, as well as your risk of developing diabetes. And these factors do increase your risk. That's why it's important to eat a diet that includes more whole-grain breads, cereals, grains, fruits, and vegetables, with moderate amounts of low-fat milk and meat products.

Be sure to choose low-salt, unsalted, or "reduced

sodium'' versions of processed foods like snacks and crackers, soups, canned and frozen vegetables, and prepared entrees. Most people eat too much salt. In some people, that can lead to high blood pressure.

 ## A Heart-Healthy Eating Plan

The basic food groups needed for a healthy heart are described below in detail. We've included the number of servings you need every day from each food group. Even if you eat the lowest number of servings listed, you will get enough protein, vitamins, and minerals. If you don't need to lose weight, or if you wish to gain weight, choose more servings from the breads and cereals and fruits and vegetables groups.

This plan from the American Heart Association is appropriate for all healthy people two years of age and older. Growing children and teenagers have special needs for calories and nutrients. If you (or others in your family) are pregnant or breast-feeding, or have a medical disorder such as diabetes, you have special dietary needs. Talk to your doctor, a Registered Dietitian, licensed dietitian, or licensed nutritionist about your diet.

Breads, Cereals, Pastas, and Starchy Vegetables

The foundation of a healthful diet is the breads, cereals, pastas, and starchy vegetables group. These foods are usually low in fat and cholesterol and are excellent sources of complex carbohydrates, fiber, vitamins, and iron. Examples of foods from this group are:

Bread
English muffins

Tortillas
Bagels
Ready-to-eat cereal
Hot cereal
Rice
Pasta (except those made with egg yolk)
Animal or graham crackers
Pretzels (unsalted)
Fig bar or ginger snap cookies
Soda or saltine crackers
Potatoes, corn, green peas, and other starchy vege-
    tables

The recommended number of servings per day is six or more. This is the minimum amount appropriate for a child, inactive woman, or someone trying to lose weight. Teenagers, men, and people who are physically active will need to eat more servings from this group depending on their total caloric expenditure.

Kendall was trying to get at least six servings of the breads group in his daily diet. He started off with two pieces of toast in the morning and had two doughnuts at his break. At lunch he ordered what he thought was a "healthful" lunch—chicken salad on a croissant. Kendall was stunned when he discovered that doughnuts and croissants are part of the desserts and sweets group! ●

Most foods in the breads, cereals, pastas, and starchy vegetables group are low in fat. But too often, people add fats to these otherwise low-fat foods. The table below describes typical high-fat additions and low-fat alternatives.

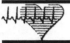 **HIGH-FAT VS. LOW-FAT ADDITIONS**

Food	Typical Additions	Low-Fat Alternatives
Bread, Toast, and Rolls	Butter or margarine	Jelly or jam
Pasta	Creamy cheese sauces	Marinara and red sauces
Hot and Cold Cereals	Whole milk	Skim milk
Baked Potatoes	Regular sour cream	Nonfat sour cream, non-fat yogurt
Cooked Vegetables and Rice	Butter or margarine	Low-fat and nonfat dressings

While six or more servings a day may sound like a lot, it really does add up quickly. All it takes is a small bowl of cereal and a piece of toast for breakfast, a sandwich with two slices of bread at lunch, a cup of cooked rice and one-half cup of corn for supper. Each of the following amounts is equal to one serving.

1 slice bread
½ English muffin or bagel
½ hot dog or hamburger bun
1 ounce ready-to-eat cereal
½ cup cooked cereal, rice, or pasta
¼-½ cup starchy vegetables

Fruits and Vegetables

When your mother nagged you about eating your vegetables, she truly had your best interests at heart. Many vegetables are a great source of vitamins, such as vitamin A or vitamin C. They are also good sources of minerals and fiber.

Fruits are often referred to as nature's candies. They are sweet, satisfying, and many come with their own easy-to-remove "wrapper." Unlike candy, fruits pack a lot of important vitamins, fiber, and carbohydrates into their "wrappers." By themselves, fruits and vegetables contain no cholesterol (remember, cholesterol only comes from animal sources). In their natural forms, they are generally low in fat and sodium. Avocados and olives are exceptions to this low-fat rule.

To be at your healthiest, aim for at least five servings of fruits and vegetables each day. It's easy to get this amount. Simply have a small glass of orange juice for breakfast, a green salad at lunch, a piece of fruit for an afternoon snack, and two servings of vegetables for supper. A serving of vegetables is just one cup of raw, leafy greens; one-half cup of raw, chopped, or cooked vegetables; or six ounces of vegetable juice. A single fruit serving is:

a medium-size piece
¼ cup of dried fruit (raisins, apricots, prunes)
6 ounces of fruit juice

Joel will not eat anything green. He won't eat broccoli, spinach, or even green beans! The closest he will come to eating something green is pale iceberg lettuce. In fact, he only likes a couple of vegetables (potatoes and corn). Unfortunately, they more closely resemble the bread group in nutrient composition. He developed this habit as a youngster, when his mother served him vegetables that were overcooked, soggy, drenched with bacon grease, and otherwise unappealing. That experience spoiled him for a lifetime. Or did it? ●

If you're like Joel, give veggies another chance. See "Heart-Healthy Cooking," pages 99–102, for easy ways to prepare crisp, delicious vegetable dishes.

Some people complain that it's inconvenient to locate and eat fruit on a regular basis. This may have been true in the past, but today there are lots of ways to enjoy the sweet sensations of fruit.

FANTASTIC FRUIT FINDS

Convenience store refrigerators
Fresh fruit salads at salad bars
Road-side fruit stands in season
Cut up fruit in grocery store produce sections
Canned fruits packed in fruit juices
Single-serving-size containers of fruit juice to pack
   in lunches or buy at a vending machine
Fruits frozen without added sugar

Low-fat Milk, Yogurts, and Cheeses

Many adults think they can quit drinking milk or eating dairy products as soon as they finish growing in their late teens and early twenties. And many of today's children drink soft drinks instead of milk. But dairy products provide protein, vitamins, calcium, and other minerals that are essential throughout life, although the amounts vary depending on life stage.

For adults and young children (ages 2–10 years), two or more daily servings of dairy products are recommended. Women who are pregnant or breast-feeding and teenagers and young adults (ages 11–24 years) need three to four servings per day.

As Gennie Lynn got older, she was less and less able to tolerate milk. Her doctor suspected that she was becoming lactose-intolerant.

"Lactose is a naturally occurring sugar in milk," Dr. Slocum explained. "Normally, you have an enzyme called lactase in your digestive tract that breaks down lactose so it can be absorbed into the bloodstream. Low lactase means that some of the lactose is not being digested. This can lead to bloating, gas, diarrhea, and cramping. Some people have a low level of lactase from birth, although it is much more common to lose lactase as we get older. This is what has probably happened to you."

It turns out that Gennie Lynn can tolerate small amounts of milk. Cheese and yogurt don't seem to bother her since their lactose levels are lower. She also uses one of the special milk products that has lactase added to it so that much of the lactose is broken down even before it is consumed. However, to make sure she is getting enough calcium, Gennie Lynn has to pay close attention to her serving sizes. ●

Some people give up dairy products because they believe them to be high in fat and cholesterol. In fact, many of the regular versions of milk, yogurt, and cheese *are* high in total fat, saturated fat, and cholesterol.

But food manufacturers have answered consumers' pleas for lower-fat alternatives. Today there are low-fat and nonfat versions of many of your favorite items. They are also lower in saturated fat and cholesterol, yet still contain the same nutrients as the whole-milk versions. Look for milk, yogurt, and cottage cheese products made with skim or 1 percent milk. Also, try natural and processed cheeses that have five grams of fat or less per ounce.

If you are accustomed to eating whole-milk products, try to gradually switch to the lower fat versions. Here's one way to do it.

1. Combine equal parts of whole milk and 2 percent milk for a couple of weeks.
2. Then use only 2 percent milk for a couple of weeks.
3. Next, combine equal parts of 2 percent milk and 1 percent milk for several weeks.
4. Then use only 1 percent milk for a couple weeks.
5. Finally, combine equal parts of 1 percent milk and skim milk for several weeks.
6. You can use this combination all the time, or skim milk, if you desire.

Try a similar tactic for getting accustomed to lower-fat cheeses, especially when you are using cheese in recipes.

Ken is a nine-year-old boy whose parents are divorced. He lives with his mother except for two weeks in the summer when he visits his dad. On the first morning of a recent visit, Ken's dad learned abruptly that Ken had changed his way of eating. He was pouring the milk on Ken's cereal when all of a sudden Ken started screaming, "I don't like that kind of milk! I won't eat it! I won't! I won't!"

After calming Ken down, his dad glanced at the label and saw that it was 2 percent milk. "Oh, great," he thought, "I only have skim and 2 percent milk. Now I've got to go to the store and get whole milk."

Just then, Ken emphatically stated, "I only like skim milk." With a sigh of relief—and pleasantly surprised—his dad started with a new bowl of cereal and topped it off with his son's new preferred choice—skim milk. ●

Lean Meat, Poultry, Fish, Eggs, and Dry Beans

"Hey Mom, what's for dinner?" is a familiar query that is often given a one or two-word answer such as "hamburgers," "baked chicken," "beef stew," or "pork chops." For generations our culture has placed meat at the center of our plates and our diets. As we've learned more about nutrition and the importance of healthful eating to prevent disease, we realize that protein is a relatively small part of a heart-healthy diet. That's because most foods in this group are significant sources of fat, saturated fat, and cholesterol.

How much protein is enough? The AHA recommends two servings per day, figuring a serving as three ounces of cooked or four ounces raw meat, poultry, or fish. In other words, no more than six ounces of cooked lean meat, poultry, or fish per day. Examples of a three-ounce portion are:

½ chicken breast or a chicken leg with a thigh;
a serving about the size of one deck of playing cards;
a serving about the size of a woman's palm, one-half an inch thick; or
2 thin slices of lean roast beef (each slice about 3″ × 3″ × ¼″).

The recommended serving size of eggs is a little different from other foods in this group. The AHA recommends eating only three to four egg yolks per week. This includes egg yolks used in cooking, such as egg noodles and baked products. Since all of the egg's cholesterol is in its yolk, you can eat all the egg whites you want.

Studies show that people get most of their dietary fat—especially saturated fat—from the meat group. So it's a good place to target for dietary changes. Here are some simple substitutions and solutions.

• Choose lean cuts of meat. Look for "round" and "loin" in the name. Choose the "Select" or "Choice" grades instead of "Prime."

- Choose ground beef, turkey, and chicken labeled "lean" or "extra lean."
- Trim all the fat from meats, and remove the skin from poultry before cooking.
- Include fish often. Shellfish (lobster, shrimp, crayfish) is higher in cholesterol than other types of fish, but it is lower in fat than most types of meat or poultry.
- Use commercial egg substitutes or substitute two egg whites for each whole egg in cooking.
- Indulge in meatless meals several times a week. One cup of cooked dry beans (pinto, navy, kidney), peas, or lentils is a low-fat, no-cholesterol substitute for a 3-ounce serving of meat, poultry, or fish.
- Use meat as a condiment instead of the main focus of a dish. For example, use smaller amounts of beef in stews or small pieces of beef in a vegetable stir-fry.

Sal had been trying to reduce his cholesterol level for years. Finally he decided to cut back on the number of times a week he ate red meat and on his meat portion sizes. About six weeks before he was due for a medical check-up, he decided to give vegetarianism a try. Sal defined vegetarian as not eating meat, poultry, eggs, or fish. He did eat dairy products.

It was a struggle, but Sal made it through the six weeks without eating meat. He wasn't thrilled about the vegetarian eating style, although it did get easier with time. He felt he could maintain it most of the time if it helped keep his blood cholesterol level under control. Sal was stunned and disappointed when his tests showed that his blood cholesterol level not only didn't go down, it went up!

The doctor suggested that Sal talk to Carol, a dietitian, about his diet. After reviewing Sal's food records,

Carol discovered that, indeed, Sal had been faithful to his vegetarian diet. He had eaten no meat, poultry, fish, or eggs for the last six weeks. But Sal did something that's common among people who cut back on their meat intake: he dramatically increased the amount of cheese he ate. He thought he needed the cheese for protein, since he had cut out meat. So instead of having a ham and cheese sandwich, Sal would have a cheese and cheese sandwich!

Carol informed Sal that, ounce-for-ounce, most cheeses have more saturated fat than a lot of meats. So instead of reducing his saturated fat intake he had actually increased it. "That," Carol explained, "is probably why your blood cholesterol level went up." To meet his protein requirements, Carol suggested that Sal eat small portions of very lean meats, limit his cheese to low-fat and nonfat varieties, and include more beans, peas, and lentils. ●

Desserts, Sweets, and Snacks

These foods are delicious, but they offer little in the way of important nutrients and are often high in fat and calories. Thus, the recommendation is to eat them sparingly. If you have low daily calorie needs or you're trying to lose weight, you'll want to eat these foods rarely. People with higher calorie needs or who need to gain weight should still eat them sparingly.

When choosing foods from this group, here is one philosophy to keep in mind: There is no such thing as "junk" food. Not even potato chips, candy bars, or a gooey Danish qualifies. All foods, even the ones in this group, can be included as a part of a healthful diet once in awhile. *The key to maintaining a healthful diet is moderation.* If your diet is composed of foods mostly from this group, you could be eating a "junk" diet; one that is high in fat and calories but low in nutrients.

Erica had never been able to tame her "sweet tooth." Yet she was aware that she needed to lower her fat intake to lose some weight. When the new low-fat and fat-free cookies, cakes, chips, and crackers began pouring onto the market, she was ecstatic. "Finally," she thought, "I can eat sweets and still lose weight!"

After several months of including low-fat sweets in her regular diet, Erica was frustrated that she hadn't lost any weight. In fact, she had gained three pounds! In a panic, she consulted a dietitian. The dietitian explained, "Erica, you have 'Fat-Free Amnesia Syndrome.' " After studying the quizzical look on Erica's face, the dietitian smiled. "It's not really a disorder. It happens to people who eat a lot of fat-free products. They simply forget that while it may be fat-free, it's not calorie-free." Sure enough, Erica interpreted "fat-free" on the label as "eat as much as you want." So even though her fat intake decreased, her calorie intake was higher than ever. ●

Fats and Oils

All foods in this group are high in fat and calories. Therefore, it's important to choose the type of fats and oils that are best for you. Here are some ideas to put you on the right track.

- When selecting cooking oils, choose ones with no more than 2 grams of saturated fat per tablespoon. These include canola, olive, safflower, corn, sunflower, and soybean.
- Select margarines with liquid vegetable oil listed as the first ingredient. These should have no more than 2 grams of saturated fat per tablespoon.
- Choose salad dressings and mayonnaise with no

more than 1 gram of saturated fat per tablespoon. (Try the reduced-fat and fat-free versions.)
- Choose low-fat or fat-free cookies, cakes, and snack foods.
- Limit the amount of fat you add when preparing or serving foods.
- Use vegetable cooking spray to lightly grease pans.

 ## Heart-Healthy Eating Patterns: Achieving a Balance

No single food or food group can give you all the nutrients you need. That's why it is important to get a balanced diet by including foods from each of the food groups each day.

So now you know the foods you should be eating. How do you put it together for a total day?

What follows are practical suggestions for ways to increase fiber, fruits, and vegetables. These hints will also help you reduce total fat, saturated fat, cholesterol, and sodium at different mealtimes. Put a check (✓) mark beside at least three strategies you could adopt for each meal.

Breakfast—Jump Start Your Day

Breakfast is an oft-maligned meal. "I don't have time." "I get nauseous if I think about eating before noon." "I'm trying to lose weight." All of these are common reasons cited for skipping breakfast. But the morning meal is important because it literally "breaks the fast" that your body has experienced since dinner the previous evening.

Depending on when you normally eat dinner and when you have your coffee break or lunch the following day, you could be literally "starving" your body of important nutrients for twelve to sixteen hours! There is little reason to wonder why you need that second (third, fourth, or fifth) cup of coffee by late morning just to keep you going. Research suggests that people who start off the day with a low-fat meal tend to end up with a low intake of fat for the entire day.

Breakfast can be simple, quick, and nutritious. Here are several ideas to help you get going in the morning.

- Choose a low-fat, high-fiber ready-to-eat cereal. After cleaning up from dinner the night before, set the table with bowls, spoons, and cereal boxes. Use skim or 1 percent milk on your cereal, then drink a small glass of fruit juice on the way to work.
- Passengers in the car can eat ready-to-eat cereal on the way to work or school. Take along a box of juice to drink in the car. You can even bring a container of yogurt to eat when you get to work.
- Make a smoothie by whirring together nonfat vanilla yogurt and fruit in a blender. Drink it while you are getting ready, or take it with you to drink during your commute.
- Make fruit parfaits for the whole family the night before, and store them in the refrigerator for an instant meal. Alternate layers of cut up fresh or canned fruit with the nonfat yogurt of your choice. Enjoy with a low-fat muffin or toast with jam.
- Pop low-fat frozen waffles in the toaster and top with mashed fruit.

Who says you have to eat traditional breakfast food in the morning? Here are some great—if somewhat unconventional—ideas for quick breakfasts.

- Zap a couple of slices of cold, veggie pizza in the microwave for a few seconds.
- Try a toasted English muffin with a twist. Top it off with low-fat cottage cheese and a tablespoon of your favorite jam, then broil it lightly.
- Skip the fat-laden breakfast sandwiches offered by fast food outlets. Make your own from low-fat cheese, lean ham or Canadian bacon, bread, bagel, or English muffin.
- Consider leftovers. All they may need is simple reheating and you have a quick breakfast.

Many people think they don't have time for breakfast. Here are some time-saving strategies for even the most rushed mornings.

- After you've eaten, rinse the dishes and leave them for a more thorough washing later when you do the dinner meal dishes.
- Choose a simple meal. Save French toast, homemade pancakes, and other more elaborate dishes for the weekends when you have more time.

Lunch—
Take Control of Your Midday Meal

Brown bag it, if you can. That way you have control over what goes into the food you eat.

- Pack your lunch for the next day while you are cleaning up from dinner. Put leftovers in microwave-safe containers.
- Spend your lunch hour once a week stocking up on lunch meals you can keep in the refrigerator/freezer at work. Suggested items include:
    A quart of skim or 1 percent milk,
    Several cartons of nonfat yogurt,
    Fresh fruit,
    Vegetable pieces and low-fat dressing or dip,

Fruit juices,
Low-fat cheeses, and
Low-fat frozen entrees and meals.
- Keep your desk stocked with heart-healthy items in case you forget your lunch or can't get away from your office. Then you won't be at the mercy of the vending machines! Try:
  Fruit juices in aseptic paper packages,
  Boxes of ready-to-eat cereal,
  Low-fat crackers and cookies,
  Dried fruit, and
  Individual portion-size cans of tuna.
- If you do eat out for lunch, try walking to a nearby restaurant. Not only do your legs get a chance to stretch but so does your heart! Check "Fueling Up at the Pump: Eating Away from Home," pages 102–108, for tips on making heart-healthy choices when eating out.

Snacks—
Treat Yourself with Healthy Choices

"Don't eat between meals, it will spoil your appetite!" How many times did you hear that when you were a kid? Perhaps you have repeated it to your own kids.

Snacking has gotten a bad rap mostly because of the foods that are typically associated with snacking. Think of what's in the "snack foods" aisle at your local supermarket: soft drinks, high-fat chips and crackers, dips, candy bars, etc. But eating between meals can be an important part of a heart-healthy diet, especially with our "on the go" lifestyles.

For example, if you go too long between meals, your blood sugar level will drop to the point where you begin to feel hungry. If you ignore the hunger sensation ("I have to pick the kids up at soccer practice before I can start dinner"), your blood sugar will drop even further. You may begin to feel anxious, get a headache, or feel lightheaded. Eating a piece of fruit, low-fat crackers, or nonfat yogurt can quickly stabilize your blood sugar level.

Also, many people who eat low-fat meals often find themselves feeling hungry well before the next meal. Low-fat meals simply take less time to digest than higher-fat meals. So you may need easy access to heart-healthy snacks such as:

- Low-fat crackers and cookies;
- Fruit (fresh, canned in fruit juice, dried, or frozen);
- Skim milk or low-fat and nonfat yogurt;
- Bagels, whole-grain breads, low-fat muffins; and
- Low-fat or nonfat cheeses.

You can find at least one of these items at nearly any convenience store, and supermarkets will certainly carry them. Or simply save a piece of fruit from a meal for a snack later in the day.

Dinner—Keep It Simple and Tasty

People rarely sit down to an evening meal at home any more. Parents work long hours and kids are busy with sports practices or school functions. With more women in the workforce, no one is at home making an elaborate meal for dinner. So to fit with today's lifestyles, the evening meal needs to be simple and fast as well as nutritious. Too big a bill to fill? Not if you use a base of good sense, add a pinch of creativity and a dash of adventure! Here are some ideas to help make dinner simple, fast, and heart-healthy.

- When the members of your family are old enough, have them choose one night a week to be in charge of dinner. Have them read the nutrition sections of this book, and keep several heart-healthy cookbooks on hand to help guide them.

- If you live alone, get together often with your circle of friends for heart-healthy potluck meals. No one gets stuck with making the entire meal and everyone gets a chance to try new heart-healthy recipes. You can even make a rule that the host/hostess gets to keep the leftovers! Try different theme nights and recipe exchanges to learn new ways for preparing foods that are low in fat, saturated fat, cholesterol, and sodium.

- Try a K.I.S.S.—Keep It a Simple Supper. Use bread, whole grains, pasta, and starchy vegetables as the base of the meal. Add low-fat ingredients or toppings. Serve with a green salad and a glass of skim milk for a balanced meal.

  Stuff a baked potato with veggies or leftover turkey chili, and then sprinkle it with low-fat cheese.

  Top an uncooked pizza shell with low-sodium tomato sauce, a little part-skim or nonfat mozzarella, and lots of veggies!

  When boiling pasta, throw in lots of frozen vegetables during the last few minutes; drain pasta and veggies; put mixture back in saucepan, add a low-fat tomato sauce, and heat thoroughly. It's a hearty, healthy entree all in one pot!

  Boil up a big batch of rice. Freeze one-half for a convenient ingredient in future meals. Stir up a quick stir fry of skinless chicken breast and lots of veggies. Serve over the cooked rice.

- Who has the time to cook from scratch any more? The good news is you don't have to. Take advantage of the many new products on the market to help make mealtime less hectic.

Try the low-fat simmering sauces for chicken.

Tired of chopping veggies for stir fry meals? Give the frozen prepackaged varieties a whirl. Tone down the amount of soy sauce you use and watch the amount of fat you put in the skillet or wok.

Instead of soaking and cooking dry beans and peas for hours, use canned varieties. Simply drain well and rinse off any excess salt before using in your favorite recipes.

Use prepackaged salads, but be careful of the dressing and croutons that are included in some varieties—they are high in fat.

If peeling, slicing, and chopping are too time-consuming, use frozen vegetables and fruits. Canned fruits (in fruit juice) and no-salt-added canned vegetables can also help cut down meal preparation time.

Choose a low-sodium, low-fat soup and add extra vegetables and cooked rice or pasta for a nutritious and filling meal. Perk up the flavor with your favorite herbs and spices.

 ## Kitchen Equipment— Keys to Low-Fat Cooking

Do you know someone who is skilled at maintaining and repairing auto engines? Chances are he or she would have all the tools, supplies, and replacement parts on hand needed to keep a car running smoothly. Doesn't it make sense to do the same for your body's engine—your heart?

Take time to inventory your kitchen, pantry, and cupboards. Think of it as a "pantry raid"! You might be surprised by what you find. The items included

on the checklist below are ones that you will find
particularly useful in helping you reduce the fat in
your cooking. Standard kitchen items such as measuring cups and spoons, pot holders, and cutting boards
are not on this list.

At the end of each section, identify items or ingredients that you need to throw out, use up, or restock.
If you are lacking in some of these items, you can
acquire them gradually. Dropping a few well-placed
hints at holiday or birthday time works wonders!

Indispensable Pots, Pans, and Cookers

Every help-your-heart kitchen needs the following
cooking supplies, geared to help you cook with your
heart in mind.

- *Skillets, saucepans, a large soup pot with non-
  stick coating.* The coating minimizes the amount
  of fat you need. Lids are needed for nearly
  each one.
- *Electric wok or skillet.* These tend to take longer
  to modulate temperatures than ones that use gas
  ranges, but if you don't cook with gas it's your
  only choice!
- *Crock pot.* Cooks while you are away all day.
  Great for slow cooking dry beans, stews, and
  tougher cuts of meat.
- *Microwave oven.* Chances are you already have
  one. If you don't, give some thought to getting
  one. Microwaving retains nutrients better than
  regular cooking methods. It will also save you
  time and, possibly, money on your energy bill.

Great Gadgets and Basic Essentials

You don't have to be a gourmet cook to know that
there are hundreds of kitchen gadgets to slice, dice,

chop, and separate. The ones listed below are custom-made to help you keep vitamins, minerals, and nutrients—while trimming the fat.

- *Sharp knives.* Don't rely on one small steak knife to "cut it" for all your cooking needs. You'll find cooking more enjoyable if you have at least a bread knife, a paring knife for delicate cutting jobs and trimming fat off meats, and a good-sized chef's knife. But don't go overboard for knives you'll rarely if ever use. Keep a sharp edge on your knives. That way they are easier and safer to use.

- *Garlic press.* Garlic adds so much to so many foods but mincing it with a knife can get tedious. A lot of heart-healthy recipes call for an abundance of garlic. Some garlic presses store peeled garlic cloves in the handle so all you need is to give it a quick twist. This is fine if you use garlic very frequently. Otherwise, select a sturdy hand-held press.

- *Juicer.* No, its not necessary to buy one of those expensive electric juicers. A simple hand variety is all you need to extract fresh lemon or lime juice.

- *Gravy separator.* It looks like a measuring cup but the spout comes from the bottom. This design allows you to pour out and retain the broth part of meat drippings, soups, or stews. You can easily leave behind the fat that has floated to the top.

- *Steamer rack or basket.* For range-top steaming, a simple rack that elevates vegetables over a small amount of liquid in a saucepan is all you need. For steaming in the microwave, you don't even need a rack. It's as easy as adding one or two tablespoons of water, covering the container with plastic wrap, venting it slightly, and cooking

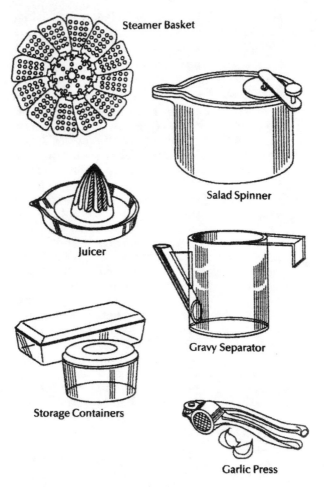

Steamer Basket

Salad Spinner

Juicer

Gravy Separator

Storage Containers

Garlic Press

FIGURE 5
Helpful Kitchen Gadgets

on high for several minutes. Most frozen vegetables do not require added water.

- *Food processor or good quality blender.* This is essential for whipping up fruit smoothies, pureeing soups, making low-fat dips from cottage cheese, etc.

- *Salad spinner.* While not essential, it's nice to have if you have room to store it. It enables you to wash salad greens and have them ready for a salad in seconds. Say good-bye to soggy greens, pat drying lettuce, or waiting for leaves to air-dry.

- *Storage containers.* Have lots of different sizes on hand for leftovers and bulk cooking. Be sure to include some that can go directly from the freezer to the microwave.

- *Covered casserole dishes.* These are great for making "one pot" entrees or meals. Have several different sizes on hand.

- *Heart-healthy cookbooks.* All you need is one or two good books to open up a whole new world of heart-healthy possibilities. Review books first to make sure the types of recipes included will be appealing to you and your family.

Heart-Healthy Ingredients

If you don't have the necessary ingredients on hand, you can't expect to cook in a heart-healthy way. Our list doesn't include basic ingredients like flour, sugar, fresh garlic, onions, potatoes, carrots, etc. Instead, we've listed ingredients that will help you achieve a lower-fat diet.

CUPBOARD CLOSE-UP. A critical part of heart-healthy cooking is packing your cupboard with things you can cook with instead of fat. Here are a few items you'll want to keep on hand to add flavor instead of fat and calories.

- *Spices*. How old are the ones in your pantry? If they're too old, they lose their zest, so consider replacing them. But be sure to buy only the spices you like and use often. Include at least one type of salt-free herb seasoning mix. Review your favorite cookbooks to find out which spices are called for most frequently. Keep them in a cool, dry area. Arrange them in alphabetical order for quick access.

- *Reduced-sodium soy sauce*. This is a must for stir fries, but it's also useful in marinades and basting sauces.

- *Vinegars*. Wine, cider, and white distilled vinegars are most common, but give balsamic and the herbed varieties a try, too. They are smoother and milder than the more common vinegars.

- *Low-sodium canned broth or mix*. Broth usually comes in beef, chicken, or vegetable varieties. They all make a great base for soups and stews.

- *A variety of dry beans (pinto, kidney, garbanzo, navy, etc.)*. Beans can be served as a low-fat side dish or added to soups, chilis, and salads. If you have time, start with the dried beans and cook them according to a low-fat recipe. But keep several canned beans on hand for quick use.

- *Canned tomatoes and tomato paste*. Choose the ones without added salt, if possible. They provide a great base for pizza and pasta sauces, soups, and stews.

- *Pastas and noodles*. Have several shapes and sizes on hand to use with just about any recipe. Look for noodles that are made without egg yolks.

- *Ready-to-eat cereals*. Include high-fiber and whole grain varieties. Cereals make a great snack as well as a quick meal.
- *Rice*. Whether it's brown, white, or instant, choose the variety that best suits your cooking style.

DOES YOUR KITCHEN PASS THE REFRIGERATOR RE-VIEW? Take a look at the heart of a heart-healthy kitchen: your refrigerator. This list below covers the basics.

- *Low-fat and nonfat milk products*. How do your selections of milk, yogurt, and cheese stack up against AHA recommendations? (See pages 68–70.)
- *Margarine*. Is it a soft tub type with liquid vegetable oil listed as the first ingredient? Does it have less than two grams of saturated fat per table-spoon?
- *Fruits and vegetables*. What kind do you have? Are they fresh and useable or are they wilted, moldy, or slimy? Could you get the recommended number of servings for each group just from what you have in your refrigerator?
- *Lemons, limes, and oranges*. The first two are often used to perk up foods such as salads and fish. Grated rinds of each of these come in handy for a number of heart-healthy recipes. How many other types of fruits do you have stored in your fridge?
- *Meats, poultry, or fish*. What cuts do you have stored? Are these high or lower in fat? If high in fat, what would be better choices?
- *Eggs*. Do you have egg substitute or lots of whole eggs? (Remember, you can substitute two egg whites for one whole egg.)

- *Low-fat or fat-free salad dressings and mayonnaise*. Experiment with different salad dressings as a marinade for meats, poultry, and fish. They are also a great substitute for butter or margarine as a topping for steamed vegetables.
- *Several different types of mustard*. Mustard is virtually fat-free, and it's a great way to add a "zing" to a lot of foods.
- *Oils*. Check the labels to see if yours have less than 2 grams of saturated fat per tablespoon. If not, switch to canola, olive, corn, soybean, safflower, or sunflower oil. Since you won't be using much oil anyway, choose small bottles or store your oils in the refrigerator to prevent them from spoiling.
- *Whole-wheat flour, rolled oats, cornmeal, and wheat germ*. These whole-grain ingredients can add fiber and important nutrients to foods. Experiment with recipes that use these ingredients. If you don't use these items much and you have room, consider keeping them in your refrigerator or freezer.

FREEZER CONFESSIONS. Ah, the moment of truth. Is your freezer stocked with ice cream or frozen vegetables? Your help-your-heart eating plan will benefit from nutritious foods you take from the freezer and prepare in a jiffy.

- *Frozen vegetables (without added cream or cheese sauce)*. Keep several varieties on hand for those days you don't have time to wash, pare, and chop fresh vegetables.
- *Frozen dinners or entrees*. It never hurts to have a couple of low-fat varieties on hand for a quick meal.
- *Frozen desserts*. Nonfat frozen yogurt, ice milk,

and sherbet are good alternatives to rich ice creams. What varieties are in your freezer?

 ## Ten Smart Shopping Tips

When you go to the filling station to fuel up your car, your choices are relatively few: regular unleaded, super unleaded, supreme unleaded, and, perhaps, diesel. But when you go grocery shopping, you have thousands of different food products to choose from. How do you know what to select for a heart-healthy diet?

First, you know what you should be eating for a well-balanced, heart-healthy diet (see "AHA Fueling Recommendations," pages 58–59). You also know the reality of what you actually have in your kitchen. Now, it's time to put together a shopping list. Here's a plan for making a shopping list that you—and your heart—will love.

- Keep an ongoing shopping list posted in a convenient place in your kitchen. As soon as your supply of any item is getting low, write it down on your list. You can't have a heart-healthy diet if you run out of the necessary ingredients. Ask family members to add to the list as needed.
- Review "Kitchen Equipment—Keys to Low-Fat Cooking" starting on page 81. What did this show you needed?
- Read through any recipes you plan to use in the coming week. Identify ingredients you don't have and add them to your list.
- Before you go shopping, organize the items on your list by their location in the store (fresh meats, frozen foods, dairy, etc.). Now you're ready to shop.

Navigating supermarket temptations while still maintaining your goals for a heart-healthy diet is a big challenge. But you can do it if you follow these suggestions.

• *Shop only once a week.* You may want to replenish perishables in the middle of the week. But shopping more than a couple of times a week can cause you to buy foods you don't really need.

• *Take your list.* All your hard work toward keeping a heart-healthy ingredients list will be for nothing if you leave it on the kitchen counter. It's also a good idea to have a pen or pencil handy to cross things off the list as you add them to your cart.

• *Don't go to the supermarket when you are hungry!* You will be tempted to impulsively buy foods that are not on your list.

• *Start with a trip around the periphery of the store.* The odds are pretty good that you will find the fresh produce, bread, baked products, fresh meats, poultry, fish, and dairy products sections around the outside walls. By starting with an "outside lap" of the store you'll probably get most of what you need. Then all you have to do is go down only those aisles that contain the few remaining items on your list. Less browsing means less temptation!

• *Look for opportunities to try new products that are low in fat, saturated fat, cholesterol, and/or sodium.* Use discount coupons to find out how you and your family like the new products.

• *Read food labels!* Food packages are now loaded with information about what's inside (see "Food Labels—Your Road Map to Healthful Food Choices" on the next few pages). Review and compare products each time you shop, and soon you'll be label able!

● Serge and Julie were young newlyweds. They were married a couple of months after they graduated from college where they had lived in campus dormitories all four years. Except for college, neither had lived away from home. Settling into a new apartment, grocery shopping, and preparing their own meals were new experiences.

Food shopping proved to be particularly difficult. Serge and Julie were constantly spending beyond their grocery budget. When they examined their shopping habits, several patterns emerged. First, they were going to the store three or four times a week, which meant they were three or four times more likely to be tempted to buy things they didn't need. Also, they usually shopped after work, which meant they were often hungry. The hunger made it more difficult to resist impulse buying.

Finally, they rarely prepared a shopping list. So each time they went to the store, they would "roam" the aisles until the sight of a product would remind them that they needed it. When Serge and Julie realized what they were doing and changed their wayward shopping tactics, they were able to shop more efficiently and inexpensively. ●

Food Labels— Your Road Map to Healthful Food Choices

Imagine you're about to drive across the country. But when you look at your road map, you notice it was printed in 1930. How successful do you think your trip would be if you had to use this map? At the very least, you would be confused and frustrated.

For many people, the same was true for reading and understanding the labels on packaged food. As a result federal legislation was enacted in recent years to change the way food manufacturers package their products. The goal was to provide consumers with an updated and standardized "map." This will help them understand what's in packaged foods so they can attain their health goals. You can now rest assured that today's packaged food labels mean just what they say. Here is what's new on food labels:

SEEING THROUGH FALSE HEALTH CLAIMS. In the past, certain food manufacturers made claims that their food product (or a component in their food product) could provide specific health benefits. The government now regulates what kind of claims food manufacturers can make. The following health claims are based on well-established nutrient-disease connections. For example:

To Make Health Claims About	The Food Must Be
Heart disease and fats	Low in fat, saturated fat, and cholesterol
Blood pressure and sodium	Low in sodium
Heart disease and fruits, vegetables, and grain products	A fruit, vegetable, or grain product that is low in fat, saturated fat, and cholesterol and that contains at least 0.6 grams of soluble fiber, without fortification, per serving

STANDARDIZED SERVING SIZES. When reading the old labels, there seemed to be a big difference in the nutrient content of similar products. Why? Because one of the manufacturers simply based the food's nutrient breakdown on a smaller portion size. This made the product seem as if it contained less fat, when it actually didn't. The new labeling laws prevent this by standardizing portion sizes for each food based on the amount people usually eat.

NUTRIENT DESCRIPTORS. On today's packaging, when you read "fat free," "low in sodium," or "light," you can trust the description. In fact, these nutrient descriptors can only be used if a food meets strict, standardized regulations set by the government.

Nutrient Descriptor	What It Means
Light (lite)	⅓ less calories or no more than ½ the fat of the higher-calorie, higher-fat version; or no more than ½ the sodium of the higher-sodium version
Cholesterol free	Less than 2 milligrams of cholesterol and 2 grams (or less) of saturated fat per serving
Low-fat	3 grams of fat (or less) per serving
Fat-free	Less than 0.5 grams of fat per serving
Reduced-sodium	At least 25 percent less sodium per serving
Lean	Less than 10 grams of fat, 4 grams of saturated fat, and 95 milligrams of cholesterol per serving
Extra lean	Less than 5 grams of fat, 2 grams of saturated fat, and 95 milligrams of cholesterol per serving

There are many more descriptors that are allowed on food labels. The important thing to remember is now you can have confidence in what the labels are promising.

EXPANDED INGREDIENT LISTS. Ingredients are still listed in descending order of predominance (by weight) on a package label. But the list has been expanded to include food colors and other additives to provide the consumer with more detailed information.

PUTTING NUTRITION FACTS TO WORK. By far the most noticeable change in food labels is the "Nutrition Facts" label, as you can see in Figure 6, on the next page.

Companies are now required to use this format to list the nutrient content of one serving of the food contained in the package. However, certain variations are allowed if the food is not a significant source of specific nutrients or the graphic format will not fit on the package.

There are two major parts of this label. The top portion is nutrient information for a single serving of the food. This is different depending on the food. The bottom portion gives information about the Daily Values, the current public health recommendations for a person who needs 2,000 calories a day.

The Nutrition Facts Label. The new nutrition facts food label offers everything you need to plan heart-healthy meals. Put it to work for you in the following ways.

• *Use it to identify one serving size.* Does one of your typical servings of the product match up with what is listed on the label? You could use this to help you control your portion sizes for certain foods. Serving size information is listed in house-

Nutrition Facts

Serving Size ½ cup (114g)
Servings Per Container 4

Amount Per Serving

Calories 90   Calories from Fat 30

% Daily Value*

Total Fat 3g	**5%**
Saturated Fat 0g	**0%**
Cholesterol 0mg	**0%**
Sodium 300mg	**13%**
Total Carbohydrate 13g	**4%**
Dietary Fiber 3g	**12%**
Sugars 3g	
Protein 3g	

Vitamin A	80%	Vitamin C	60%
Calcium	4%	Iron	4%

*Percent Daily Values are based on a 2,000
calorie diet. Your daily values may be higher or
lower depending on your calorie needs:

	Calories	2,000	2,500
Total Fat	Less than	65g	80g
Sat Fat	Less than	20g	25g
Cholesterol	Less than	300mg	300mg
Sodium	Less than	2,400mg	2,400mg
Total Carbohydrate		300g	375g
·Fiber		25g	30g

Calories per gram:
Fat 9   •   Carbohydrate 4   •   Protein 4

FIGURE 6
Nutrition Facts Label

hold measures (½ cup), units (6 pieces, 1 slice), and gram weights.

Please note: The serving sizes on food labels don't always match up with the serving sizes given in the USDA's Food Guide Pyramid.

Walter enjoyed eating ice cream but his doctor suggested that he limit his portion size to one serving. The problem was that one of "Walter's servings" was five times the amount defined on the Nutrition Facts label! ●

- *Plan how much of a product you will need.* The servings per container information will help you decide if you need more than one package to feed your entire family.
- *Keep track of calories.* On the top of the label, this lists the amount of total calories and calories coming from fat in a single serving. If you eat two servings, you need to double this amount. Some people like to figure out the percentage of calories in a product that come from fat. You can do this by dividing the number given for calories from fat by the number given for total calories.
- *Identify nutrient composition.* The nutrients listed in Figure 6 are the ones you're going to see most often. That's because these are the ones in which most people today have an interest. Manufacturers may also include information about other nutrients, such as riboflavin, niacin, potassium, etc., but that is optional.

Nutrient Content Information. The food label also gives you a lot of information about nutrient content. When you learn how to use this information, you'll be a knowledgeable label reader.

- *Use it to track the amounts of different nutrients you consume each day.* If you're trying to cut down on fats, saturated fats, dietary cholesterol, and sodium, it's helpful to monitor your intake of these nutrients. The table below shows nutrient goals for different calorie levels. Decide which calorie level is best for you. Then track your food intake for several days using copies of the form provided in Appendix A to see if you are meeting the goals.

Food Component	DIETARY GOALS FOR DIFFERENT CALORIE LEVELS*						
	Calories						
	1,200	1,600	2,000	2,200	2,500	2,800	3,200
Total fat (g)	<40	<53	<65	<73	<80	<93	<107
Saturated fat (g)	<13	<18	<20	<24	<28	<31	<36
Dietary cholesterol (mg)	<300	<300	<300	<300	<300	<300	<300
Sodium (mg)**	<3,000	<3,000	<3,000	<3,000	<3,000	<3,000	<3,000
Dietary fiber	20	20	25	25	30	32	37

* Numbers may be rounded.
**This is the American Heart Association's sodium recommendation. The reference value for sodium listed on food labels is slightly less (no more than 2,400 milligrams per day).

- *Use the Percent Daily Value numbers as a quick way to judge whether or not a food is high in a particular ingredient.* For example, a food lists a Percent Daily Value for total fat of 50 percent. That means one serving of that particular food supplies one-half of the total daily amount of fat for a person who needs 2,000 calories. That's a lot of fat in one food item.

You can also use the Percent Daily Value numbers to quickly compare similar products. If you are looking at total fat, saturated fat, cholesterol, and sodium for similar products, choose the one that has a lower number for these nutrients.

You may have noticed that not all foods have nutrition labels. Some exceptions include:

Restaurant foods,

Foods produced by small businesses, and

Foods prepared on-site in grocery store bakery or deli departments.

Most processed meats and poultry foods will carry a nutrition label. Stores are being asked to voluntarily offer nutrition information for fresh, raw meats and poultry. Look for information cards in the fresh meat section. Similarly, some stores provide nutrition information directly or at the point of selection on raw fruits, vegetables, and fish or at the point of sale. This is voluntary for now. However, if most supermarkets neglect to include this information, the government will make labeling of these products mandatory.

The current labels were designed to help you, the health-conscious consumer, make informed food choices. Think of label reading as a skill similar to using a map. Once you know what the numbers and symbols mean, you can easily navigate your way around high-fat potholes to reach your destination of a lifetime of heart-healthy eating.

Heart-Healthy Cooking

You have stocked your kitchen with heart-healthy tools and supplies. A trip to the supermarket yields a bountiful supply of low-fat ingredients. There is only one thing left to do—start cooking!

For many people, the thought of cooking is not very appealing. For some, it's downright scary. Much of the concern comes from the feeling that you don't have time to cook. Not knowing how to prepare heart-healthy foods that taste good is another roadblock. This section will give you hints and tips that should help move you from the ranks of the "kitchen-challenged" to the "kitchen-capable."

BEFORE YOU START COOKING. Start by using recipes that are low in fat, saturated fat, and cholesterol. You can find many cookbooks (several by the American Heart Association) and magazines that specifically offer heart-healthy recipes (see Appendix B). Or modify your family favorites. To modify a recipe, ask yourself two questions:

1. *Is every ingredient necessary?* Things like nuts, olives, extra cheese, whipped toppings, and oil for basting can often be eliminated without affecting the final product significantly.
2. *If it is necessary, how can I make it more healthful?*
   - First, use less of it. Most fats and sugars can be reduced by one-quarter to one-third without drastically altering the taste.
   - Substitute a healthier version. Take your cue from the "Substitution Table" on the next page.

HEALTHY SUBSTITUTION TABLE

When your recipe calls for:	Use:
Whole milk	Skim, ½ percent or 1 percent milk
Butter	Soft (tub) margarine with liquid vegetable oil listed as the first ingredient and with less than 2 grams of saturated fat per tablespoon, or vegetable oil with less than 2 grams of saturated fat per tablespoon. Remember: 1 tablespoon butter = 1 tablespoon margarine = ¾ tablespoon oil. Use vegetable cooking spray to lightly grease skillets and pans.
Eggs	Cholesterol-free commercial egg products. Or use 2 egg whites for every whole egg.
Sour cream	Nonfat sour cream products. Or make your own by blending 1 cup low-fat cottage cheese or part-skim ricotta cheese with 1 tablespoon lemon juice.
Cheese	Low-fat or nonfat varieties (less than 3 grams of fat per ounce). Or try using less of the whole-milk variety.
Ground beef	Ground beef that is labeled "lean" or "extra lean".
Unsweetened baking chocolate	Unsweetened cocoa powder blended with unsaturated oil or margarine (3 tablespoons of cocoa powder plus 1 tablespoon of acceptable vegetable oil or margarine = one 1-ounce square of chocolate).

Modifying recipes doesn't always mean cutting back on ingredients. You can add extra vegetables and beans to soups, stews, chilis, and casseroles to "dilute" the fats and cholesterol.

When you have selected your recipes and modified them as necessary, here are a few more helpful hints you'll want to try before cooking.

- Review the recipes and assemble all the ingredients and utensils you need, except any items that should be refrigerated.
- Thoroughly wash produce and prepare as directed.
- Do all the peeling, slicing, and chopping for the recipes. This will save time.
- Trim visible fat from meats and remove the skin from poultry.

WHEN COOKING. Now for the fun part—cooking! Heart-healthy cooking does not have to be time-consuming or difficult. All you need to know are a few simple tricks of the trade. Here are a few to get you started.

- Select a low-fat cooking method such as: baking, steaming, roasting, poaching, stir-frying, broiling, braising, stewing, or grilling. See, you are not stuck with steamed food for the rest of your life!
- The usual method of sauteing vegetables in butter or oil is high in fat. Try spraying a non-stick pan with vegetable spray and adding a small amount of broth to keep the vegetables from burning or sticking.
- When baking, substitute mashed or pureed fruit (like applesauce or prunes) for some of the fat called for in the recipe.
- Use spices, herbs, and other low-salt seasonings

to perk up your menu. Experiment with different varieties on your meats, poultry, fish, and vegetables.

AFTER COOKING. When you're finished cooking, take a little more time to make sure your dishes are their heart-healthiest before serving them.

- Transfer meat drippings to a fat-separating measuring cup. If you have a plastic version, be sure to wait until the liquid cools so it doesn't melt the plastic. You may also refrigerate the drippings and remove the congealed fat when it has cooled. Use the stock for soups, low-fat gravies, and sauces.
- Put cooked ground beef or ground turkey in a colander and rinse with hot water to remove excess fat. Pat dry with paper towels before adding to a recipe such as spaghetti sauce, chili, or sloppy joes.

 ## Fueling Up at the Pump: Eating Away from Home

Even a couple of decades ago, eating out was a rare treat. Today, it's an ordinary part of everyday life. In fact, estimates show that by the turn of the century, most of the money we spend on food will be used to buy meals prepared outside of the home!

Yet eating out can be hazardous to your health. When you let a fast-order cook or a chef prepare a meal for you, you are placing your dietary health in someone else's hands. You lose control over what goes into your food.

Even so, there are things you can do to ensure that eating out doesn't do you in. Start by identifying your eating out patterns. The following three-part quiz will pinpoint where you need help. Then you can develop strategies to prepare yourself for eating out. Finally, you'll know how and what to ask for when selecting food at a restaurant. These skills will put you back in the driver's seat.

EATING AWAY FROM HOME QUIZ—PART I

On average, how many times per week do you eat the following meals away from home? (Circle one number for each meal.)

Breakfast	0	1	2	3	4	5	6	7	
Lunch	0	1	2	3	4	5	6	7	
Dinner	0	1	2	3	4	5	6	7	
Snacks	0	1	2	3	4	5	6	7	8

TOTAL number of times you eat out per week = _____

The more times per week you eat out, the more you are "at risk" for eating high-fat meals. Consequently, you'll have to pay close attention to what you're eating when dining out. How can you improve your odds? First, assess why you eat out so frequently. Then problem-solve heart-healthy solutions. For example:

Problem: Business breakfasts, lunches, dinners

Solution: Meet at a conference center or board-room. Hold the meeting somewhere besides a restaurant. Meet at a local park or the zoo and walk while you talk. If this is not possible, choose a restaurant that you know offers heart-healthy meal options.

Problem: Catered meals and breaks at work

Solution: Ask if the caterer can provide low-fat alternatives (such as bagels instead of doughnuts).

If not, suggest that your company switch to a vendor that can. Meanwhile, why not bring your own bagels and share the low-fat benefits with your colleagues.

Problem: "I don't know how to cook." or "I don't like to cook."

Solution: Expand your skills. Take a fun cooking course at the local community college. Buy a few heart-healthy cookbooks and magazines (or dust off the ones you have). Start a heart-healthy cooking club with friends. It's a great way to socialize. try new recipes, and develop new skills.

Problem: "I don't have time to cook."

Solution: Many people today live in overdrive. Still, there are ways to eat healthfully and quickly. Plan ahead. When you do cook, make a double batch so you can quickly reheat the leftovers for another meal. Look for other ideas in the section, "Heart-Healthy Eating Patterns—Achieving a Balance," pages 75–81.

If you eat out a lot more at one meal, find out why. Lunchtime is often when most people rack up most of their eating out time.

Collin ate out every lunch during the week. He had a schedule that he followed faithfully. On Monday he went to Chez Max, a popular lunch spot that was known for its smorgasbord of salads and generous servings. He ate Chez Max crab salad, Caesar salad, potato salad, and marinated vegetables. He ate the leftovers on Tuesday and Wednesday. On Thursday, Collin ate Chinese food—he always ordered sweet and sour chicken. He saved the leftovers for lunch on Friday.

Collin deserved a pat on the back for making some attempt at limiting his portion sizes by making two restaurant meals last all week. But the actual foods he chose were high in fat, saturated fat, cholesterol, and sodium. So even though his meals were smaller than if he had eaten out at different restaurants each day, he was still eating high-fat foods all week long. ●

 EATING AWAY FROM HOME QUIZ—PART II

Select the kind of restaurants or food sources you patronize at least twice a month. (Circle all that apply.)

1. Cafeteria
2. Fast-food restaurants
3. Airlines
4. Vending machines
5. Heart-healthy restaurants
6. Sporting events, movie theaters, parties
7. Family-style or full-service restaurants
8. All-you-can-eat places
9. Grocery store
10. Take-out or home-delivered food

Add together the:
Number of odd-numbered options selected = _____
Number of even-numbered options selected = _____

The odd-numbered restaurants or food sources are ones that typically make it easier for you to make heart-healthy choices.

- They offer a variety of options. These places are better choices than places that only serve fried foods, where your only choice will be a high-fat meal.

- They usually prepare food to order. In the case of airline food, you can call ahead to order special, low-fat, low-cholesterol meals. Most airlines request a 24-hour notice.
- They let you order a la carte. You can order what you want without all the extras that can add a lot of fat and calories.

The even-numbered restaurants in this list often restrict your heart-healthy options. That doesn't mean you shouldn't patronize these places. It just means that you may want to frequent them less often. Be aware that you'll have to look harder for heart-healthy selections in these establishments.

 EATING AWAY FROM HOME QUIZ—PART III

Circle the appropriate response. Be honest with yourself!

1. I usually leave food on my plate even though I know I have paid for it.	YES	NO
2. I eat out mostly just on special occasions (birthdays, anniversaries, celebrations)	YES	NO
3. I usually can find at least one heart-healthy entree at most restaurants.	YES	NO
4. I very often ask the waitstaff questions about menu items and how they are prepared.	YES	NO
5. When I go to all-you-can-eat places, I only fill my plate once.	YES	NO
6. I find myself frequently asking for a "doggie bag" to take leftovers home.	YES	NO
7. I can tell whether or not a menu item is heart-healthy by the way it is described.	YES	NO
8. I try to slow my eating by keeping pace with the slowest eater at the table.	YES	NO

9. I am aware of when I get full and then
   immediately stop eating.   YES   NO

10. I usually ask for dressings and sauces to be
    served "on the side."   YES   NO

Total number of YES responses = _____

IF YOU SELECTED

8–10 YES responses   CONGRATULATIONS!
                        You are a confident and
                        skilled diner. Keep up the
                        good work!

4–7 YES responses   You are practicing some
                        healthful eating out skills.
                        Still, there is room for im-
                        provement.

0–3 YES responses   Eating out may present
                        problems for you unless
                        you learn more heart-
                        healthy eating out skills.
                        Look at your NO re-
                        sponses for ideas.

The ten skills cited in the above quiz can help you
put some control back into eating out. Here are some
additional ideas:

- Decide what you will order before getting to the
  restaurant. You will be less likely to be caught
  off-guard by extensive menu listings, peer pressure, or the sights and smells of the restaurant.
- Decide to do the following:
     Select either a drink before dinner or a des-
        sert, but not both.
     Eat your roll without butter. Push the butter
        dish to the other side of the table.

Select foods in their simplest forms. For
example, broiled fish is a lower-fat alternative to fried or stuffed fish.

- Don't skip meals when you are planning to eat
  out later. Your self-control will disappear if you
  arrive at a restaurant hungry.
- Be the first to order. Then you can't be swayed
  by choices made by others at your table.
- Skip the appetizer, share one with a friend, or
  enjoy steamed shrimp, broth soups, or low-fat
  salads.
- Steer clear of foods described as any of the following:

      au gratin, parmesan, escalloped, in a cheese
          sauce;
      creamed, in a cream sauce, hollandaise;
      crispy, sauteed, fried; or
      in butter sauce, buttery.

- Look for entrees that are listed as:

      broiled, grilled, or baked;
      in its own juice, in tomato sauces, in lemon
          juice or wine;
      steamed; or
      poached.

- If in doubt, ask questions.
- Enjoy your meal. Focus on the company, the
  conversation, and the pleasure of knowing you
  don't have to do the dishes!

 Eating Internationally

One of the fastest growing segments of the eating out
market is ethnic foods. Regardless of what you might
have heard, there are heart-healthy alternatives on just
about every ethnic menu.

CHINESE. When eating Chinese, skip the high-sodium soups and have the fried noodles removed from the table. They are high in fat and calories. Choose dishes that are boiled, steamed, or lightly stir-fried. Ask that they use less oil and that sauces, such as soy sauce, be served on the side. Ask them to cook without salt and monosodium glutamate (MSG). Choose steamed rice over the fried rice. Steer clear of sweet and sour dishes. They are battered and fried, then drenched in sweet sauce. Ask for extra vegetables.

FRENCH. A good rule for dining out in French restaurants is "keep it simple." Steamed mussels and a salad with dressing on the side are fine starters. Avoid French onion soup, which is usually laden with cheese and high in sodium and calories. Be wary of sauces, the heart of classic French cuisine. Hollandaise, bechamel, and béarnaise are all high in fat. Look for wine- or fruit-based sauces. Or ask for the sauce on the side.

GREEK. Most of the oil used in Greek cooking is olive oil, which is high in monounsaturated fats. While a "good" oil, it is still wise to limit it for the sake of keeping your caloric intake down. Tzatziki, an appetizer made with yogurt and cucumbers, is a good way to start a Greek meal. Hummous is a bit higher in fat, but it's still a good choice. Pita bread is low in fat. Greek salads are filling and delicious. [The feta cheese is slightly lower in fat than hard cheeses, but high in sodium.] Anchovies and olives are also high in fat or sodium, so go easy on these or skip them altogether.

For a main course, stick with dishes like plaki. That's fish that's been cooked with tomatoes, onions, and garlic. Or try shish kabob, broiled on a spit and made with beef or lamb, tomatoes, onions, and peppers. Have your entree with rice. There are a few pitfalls. Lamb has more saturated fat than beef. Phyllo dishes, which can be entrees and desserts, are very high in fat because the dough is usually layered with butter. Caviar, served in some dishes, is high in cholesterol.

INDIAN. Indian food is generally low in saturated fat, cholesterol, and calories. Its tastiness is a tribute to the creative use of spices. Many dishes use a yogurt-based curry sauce. Enjoy the salads. They are often a refreshing combination of yogurt with chopped or shredded vegetables. Tandoori chicken and fish dishes are marinated in Indian spices and roasted in a clay pot. They make a delicious and authentic meal. Ask if a small amount of margarine can be used to baste the tandoori instead of butter.

Vegetables are an important part of Indian meals. Ask that ghee, the clarified butter often used in the preparation of vegetables, be eliminated. Plain rice is often a soothing accompaniment to a spicy Indian meal. Don't forget to try the wonderful breads like papadum, chapati, and nan.

ITALIAN. To many diners, Italian food means pasta. And pastas can be heart-healthy as long as they are not filled with cheese or fatty meat or tossed with butter or cream sauces. Linguine with white or red clam sauce is a fine pasta selection. Lower-fat sauces include marsala (made with wine) and marinara (made with tomatoes, onion, and garlic). Ask for extra vegetables on the Pasta Primavera, and eat it without the cream sauce.

Consider ordering the appetizer portion of pasta as your entree—often the portions are large enough to be filling. Caesar salad sounds healthful but it is rarely a good option. Eggs, anchovies, parmesan cheese, and oily dressing are part of the recipe. Among othe' selections in Italian restaurants, simply prepared chicken and fish dishes are your best bets. Italian ices are excellent dessert choices.

JAPANESE. Although many dishes are high in sodium, Japanese cuisine is, overall, a boon to fat-conscious diners. Pickled vegetables are low in cholesterol, saturated fat, and calories. And they make a lovely introduction to traditional Japanese entrees. Acceptable entrees include one-pot meals (nabemonos) like sukiyaki, shabu-shabu, or yosenabi. Try teriyakis, especially the chicken or fish varieties. Look for the word "yaki," which means broiled. Dishes that feature tofu are especially good choices. Tofu is a soybean curd protein without cholesterol and extremely low in calories. Of course, steamed rice makes a healthful accompaniment. Avoid tempura, agemono, and katsu dishes.

MEXICAN. Beans fried in lard, lots of cheese, and fried tortilla chips cause many health-conscious diners to bypass Mexican restaurants. But if you know what you're doing, you can walk away from a "south of the border" meal in great shape. For starters, push the basket of chips to the other end of the table. Ask the waiter to bring you hot corn tortillas instead for dipping in the salsa. Gazpacho soup and bean soup are good low-fat appetizers. Salads may be a good choice, but find out about the ingredients before ordering.

Fajitas (chicken, beef, shrimp) are among the better entree choices. Whether or not tacos, enchiladas, and burritos are good choices depends on what's inside them. Skip the cheese versions; bean and chicken are better options. Ask for non-fat yogurt instead of cheese; many Mexican restaurants are starting to have it.

Eating on the Run

Few people sit down to three square meals at home or at full-service restaurants every day. More people today are becoming "grazers." They eat a little bit of food many times throughout the day. Some research suggests that this tactic may actually be a healthful alternative to the one- or two-meals-a-day pattern typical of many Americans.

In one study, subjects ate their entire daily allotment of food in three meals for two weeks. They then ate the exact amount and kind of food for another two weeks, but ate it in seventeen "snacks" spaced throughout the day. The results were interesting. Compared to the three-meal pattern, the "grazing" diet significantly reduced total blood cholesterol and LDL-cholesterol levels. However, it remains to be determined how blood cholesterol levels would respond under different conditions. What if the "grazing" pattern were maintained for a longer duration? What if the subjects were overweight? What if the nutrient composition of the diet was different?

Many of you adopt a grazing-type eating pattern on some days. Some of you may do it for its potential health benefits. For others, your lives may be too hectic to think about getting "three squares." When you do eat on the run, here are strategies to help make it heart-healthy rather than haphazard.

BE A PACK HORSE. Keep low-fat foods with you in your car, at your desk, and in the refrigerator at work.

USE VENDING MACHINES JUDICIOUSLY. Look for healthful options such as the following.

- Lite microwave popcorn
- Fig bars
- Animal crackers

- Unsalted pretzels
- Graham crackers
- Dried fruit
- Fresh fruit
- Fruit juices
- Sandwiches with low-fat ingredients
- Low-fat or nonfat yogurt or milk

Watch out for granola and trail mix. They sound "healthy," but they're often high in fat.

Lobby your employer to provide healthful options in the vending machines. You would be surprised at the number of people at work who would support your efforts.

The four o'clock snack attack hit Bill like a ton of bricks. He jangled his pocket to make sure he had change and headed down the hall. As he stood in front of the snack machine, he could hear his doctor's voice, "You really need to cut down on the amount of fat in your diet." The longer he stared at the candy bars and salty chips, the louder and more insistent the voice became.

"You're right," Bill said to no one in particular. So he scanned the machine for a low-fat alternative. But to no avail. He selected a chocolate bar and vowed to himself that he was going to ask the company to make some changes in vending.

He went directly to the vice-president of facilities. He learned that he wasn't the first employee to ask for heart-healthy food options. The vice-president gave Bill the name of the vendor. Bill and the vendor collaborated on a new vending program. Employees would have at least seven heart-healthy items in each snack machine, yet the vendor's profit would stay healthy.

Bill worked with his company to find ways to promote the new vending machine items. They found two ways to do that.

They began a frequent buyer program. By turning in the wrappers from heart-healthy foods they purchase from the vending machine, employees got discounts in the company cafeteria.

They also started a sticker program. It was designed to maintain interest after the initial promotion. The vendor randomly attached stickers describing prizes to some of the heart-healthy foods. Employees who found a sticker on their purchase won the prize described.

Bill planned to conduct a survey of employee satisfaction with the vending program in six months. ●

 ## Approach Convenience Stores with Caution

You may find yourself in convenience stores often if you do a lot of eating on the run. Convenience stores can be sources of healthful foods, if you know what to look for. Try the following.

- Bagels instead of doughnuts
- Bananas and apples instead of candy bars
- Fruit juices instead of presweetened soft drinks
- Microwaved bean burrito instead of a chili hot dog
- Low-fat yogurt and milk instead of a pimento cheese sandwich
- Ready-to-eat cereal instead of nuts
- Licorice instead of chocolate candy
- Graham crackers instead of high-fat cookies and crackers

Watch Out for the Fast Lane

Too often nowadays, "life in the fast lane" means "life in the fast food lane." When you look carefully at the nutrient composition of most fast food meals, "life in the *fat* food lane" might be more appropriate.

Fast foods are notorious for high-fat items and limited choices. Even with what seems to be a fast food outlet on every corner, it remains a fast-growing industry. Schools, hospitals, and gas stations have climbed on the bandwagon by teaming up with fast food franchises.

So, they're here to stay. Fortunately, many fast-food franchises are making efforts to give consumers a few healthier choices. Here's a partial list of what to look for.

- Sandwiches
    - Small roast beef sandwich
    - Broiled plain fish or chicken breast sandwich
    - Special low-fat hamburger without cheese
    - Regular-size hamburger
- Side orders
    - French fries (Skip them, or make it a small order and share it with a friend.)
    - Baked potato (Top it with chili or broccoli and go easy on the cheese.)
    - Salad/salad bar (Use the low-fat dressing.)
- Beverages
    - Low-fat milk
    - Fruit juice
    - Low-fat shakes
- Other
    - Pizza topped with veggies and/or Canadian bacon
    - Pancakes (Use jam instead of margarine.)
    - Cold cereal with 1 percent milk
    - Fat-free muffin

    Egg English muffin (Skip the sausage and
       biscuits.)
    Low-fat frozen yogurt

Here's a partial list of what to watch out for.

* Taco salads (They sound healthier than they
  really are.)
* "Value" meals (They are usually three items—
  hamburger, fries, and a drink—sold as one meal
  at a slight discount from those items ordered
  separately. This is a sales gimmick to get you to
  buy more than you might initially be inclined
  to do.)
* Prepackaged salad dressings (These packages
  often contain two or more servings.)

 ## Heart-Healthy Traveling Tips

Whether you're on the road for business or pleasure,
there are some strategies to help you stay on track
with your heart-healthy goals. Take a look at these
ideas, and then add some of your own.

* Book yourself into a hotel or resort that offers
  healthful dining options. Call ahead and ask the
  management to fax you copies of the menus from
  the hotel's restaurants.
* Find out if the hotel has on-site exercise facilities. Many have special arrangements with
  nearby fitness centers that allow guests to use
  the facilities for little or no charge.
* When flying, remember these tips.
  > Request a special meal. Most airlines offer at
  > least one low-fat option. Some have an
  > extensive selection from which to choose.
  > Order your special meal at the time you

make your reservations or give the airline 24 hours notice. There is no extra charge.

Skip the alcoholic beverages. They add extra calories, and alcohol is a diuretic. The air in the flight cabin is dehydrating as it is; don't make it worse. Combat dehydration and pack in some vitamins by choosing tomato juice or orange juice.

Pack heart-healthy snacks in your carry-on bag. You never know what delays or problems you might experience in your travels.

Carmen was traveling overseas on a flight that left Chicago at 5:30 p.m. After about two hours, the flight attendants began serving dinner. A few moments later, they were interrupted by an announcement from the cockpit indicating that there were mechanical problems and that the flight was being rerouted to Kennedy airport in New York.

After three hours of circling, the plane finally touched down safely, and the passengers were deplaned. It was 11:30 p.m., and none of the airport shops or restaurants were open. Knowing that the passengers had not eaten, the airline arranged for sandwiches and soft drinks. Unfortunately for Carmen, who is a vegetarian, the sandwiches were turkey and ham.

But she was prepared. She always carries food with her, and this time it paid off. A bagel, a carton of fruit juice, and a small can of tuna fish later, Carmen's flight was called. She and her fellow passengers took a brand new airplane across the Atlantic. ●

• When traveling by car, remember these tips.
  Pack a cooler with low-fat cheese, fruits, and juices, cut-up vegetables, and low-fat dip.
  Include low-fat sandwiches (turkey, lean

ham, or roast beef, etc.). Put the cooler
within easy reach.

Stop frequently to stretch, walk around, and
unwind. This will help break the monot-
ony, which may contribute to eating from
boredom.

Stay at motels that have kitchenettes so you
can cook some of your own meals.

- Don't make eating the main attraction of your
trip or vacation. Cruises are notorious for this!
But wise cruise line managers have learned that
their clients also want heart-healthy menu options. Instead of a cruise, take a biking or hiking
vacation or simply sightsee on foot. You'll come
back from your trip without a lot of extra
tonnage.

 ## Holiday Survival—Be Realistic

Holidays, parties, and special occasions can wreak
havoc with the best of eating plans. But there are ways
to combat the excesses associated with the holidays.

Make a pact with yourself to allow no more than a
two-pound weight gain from the middle of November
to the first of January. Too often we throw caution to
the wind at holiday time, gaining so many pounds that
we never fully return to our pre-holiday weight. On
the other hand, don't try to lose weight during the
holidays. You'll be setting yourself up for failure and
disappointment.

MAINTAIN OR INCREASE YOUR PHYSICAL ACTIVITY. "I'm
so stressed out because of all I have to do—the last
thing I have time for is exercise!" Sound familiar?
Build physical activity into your holiday shopping by

walking briskly around the mall before you are loaded down with packages. Or spend less time shopping by using mail-order catalogs. Start a "Turkey Trot" tradition in your family—everyone has to get outside to walk before or after the holiday meal. Spend time with family or friends doing active things. Try walking, jogging, skiing, skating, dancing, etc. instead of sitting around talking. Remember, physical activity is a great stress reliever!

LOOK FOR LOW-FAT VERSIONS. Check the food sections of your local paper or heart-healthy cookbooks for recipes. Or modify your own recipes (see "Heart-Healthy Cooking," pages 99–102). Eat low-fat while at home as much as possible so that you can give yourself a little more freedom at holiday parties.

SHARE THE WEALTH. If you are inundated with gifts of food, spread around the extra fat and calories by giving some of the goodies away to charitable groups, church groups, food banks, or homeless shelters. You can also divide the food gifts into smaller amounts and freeze for later use. As a health-conscious gift-giver, practice what you preach with low-fat food gifts. Try these suggestions.

- Fruit baskets (hold the cheese unless it is a low-fat variety)
- An assortment of different pastas or rices
- Mulling spices for making hot spiced cider
- Inexpensive but essential cooking gadgets (see "Great Gadgets and Basic Essentials," pages 82–85)

Consider non-food gifts such as the ones listed below.

- Subscriptions to low-fat cooking magazines
- Gift certificate for a massage

- Books
- A pedometer
- Running shoes

BE A HEART-HEALTHY HOST/HOSTESS. When it's your turn to "put on a spread," offer low-fat options. If your guests are new to heart-healthy eating or might be a bit squeamish about such food, simply don't tell them it's heart-healthy.

USE HEART-HEALTHY PARTY TACTICS. Eat something at home before you go to a party so you are not "starving" when you arrive. Always hold a glass of seltzer water or diet soft drink in one hand. It's hard to eat a plateful of food when you're holding a drink. If you do drink alcoholic beverages, alternate one alcoholic beverage with a low-calorie, non-alcoholic drink. Navigate your way around the party so that you are not constantly standing at the buffet table. Instead of eating, spend your time socializing with friends and family. After all, that's why you were invited!

 Where to Get More Nutrition Help

This section of the book has given you general information about nutrition as it relates to heart health. We've also given you practical tips for making changes that can help you reduce your fat, saturated fat, cholesterol, and sodium intakes.

If you want additional help personalizing these recommendations, seek the advice of a nutrition counselor. He or she can tailor a program to meet your particular medical needs, daily habits, or personal preferences. Look for a Registered Dietitian, Licensed Dietitian, or Licensed Nutritionist. These professionals are highly qualified to help you follow your doctor's dietary prescription and to counsel you effectively.

The letters "R.D." after a name stand for Registered Dietitian. That means the nutritionist has been certified by the American Dietetic Association. An R.D. must have completed a bachelor's degree, with an emphasis on food and nutrition, and an approved internship. He or she must also have passed a national examination. Licensed Dietitians ("L.D") and Licensed Nutritionists ("L.N.") also have degrees in food science or nutrition and are licensed by the state in which they work. Each state has its own licensing requirements.

If you think you would benefit from the advice and guidance that a nutrition expert could provide, ask your doctor for a referral. In fact, many nutrition counselors only accept those people who have been referred by physicians. If your doctor cannot recommend anyone, there are still ways to find a good nutrition counselor.

- Some hospital outpatient clinics offer nutrition counseling for specific disease conditions. Your physician can probably tell you about those available in your area.
- Check the yellow pages of your phone book under Health Care Services, Dietitians, Nutritionists. Contact the American Dietetic Association or your state Dietetic Association.
- Call your local Public Health Department.
- Call the nutrition department of your local university.

Remember that dietary change takes time. Together, you and your nutrition counselor can plan a schedule to help you make changes slowly. Think of your dietitian or nutrition counselor as a guide leading you toward a goal of improved health. It's up to you to follow the instructions and advice your counselor provides. And the success of your new eating plan is in your hands. Good luck!

 Facts and Fallacies About Nutrition

I am trying to cut out all fat in my diet. Will that harm me?

Yes, it will definitely harm you. Don't even consider doing it. The truth is, at least 1 to 2 percent of your daily calories should come from fat (compared to the national average of 34 percent). It must be in the form of linoleic acid. This is a fatty acid that the body cannot make, and thus must be obtained in the diet, mostly from vegetable oils. Also, you need some fat to help absorb fat-soluble vitamins from the intestine.

Fortunately, it would be nearly impossible to cut your fat intake to 1 percent unless you ate a diet that severely restricted many of the food groups. Even a well-balanced all-vegetarian diet will give you moderate amounts of fat from grain products, legumes, and some vegetables.

For good health, aim for a balanced, nutritious diet that includes all the food groups, but is low in total fat, saturated fat, cholesterol, and sodium.

Saturated fats only come from animal products, right?

Wrong. Fatty meats and whole-milk dairy products are indeed high in saturated fatty acids. But so are palm, palm kernel, and coconut oils, which come from plants. Saturated fat from animals tends to be solid at room temperature. Plant sources of saturated fats are liquid at room temperature.

I switched from butter to margarine years ago, but now I hear that margarine is bad for me. Can I go back to butter?

From what we know today, margarine is still better than butter. The issue that brought the butter-margarine controversy to a fever pitch is trans fatty acids (TFAs). To make margarine, vegetable oil undergoes a process called hydrogenation. Hydrogenation makes the oil more saturated with hydrogen atoms (hence the name) and thus more solid at room temperature (like butter). It also creates TFAs, a type of fatty acid not found in nature. Some studies have suggested that TFAs increase low-density lipoprotein (LDL) cholesterol as much as butter. LDL cholesterol is often called the "bad" cholesterol, because it tends to attach to the lining of the arteries.

We know that butter definitely contains large amounts of both saturated fat and cholesterol. For that reason, we still recommend margarine. Choose a tub-type margarine where the first ingredient listed is liquid vegetable oil and that contains no more than 2 grams of saturated fat per tablespoon.

The important thing to remember is to use small amounts of any fat, be it margarine or vegetable oil.

A friend of mine is taking fish oil pills to "protect his heart." Does he know something I don't?

Your friend has probably read about the studies that indicated that the type of oils found in fatty fish reduces blood cholesterol levels. Since those studies surfaced, enterprising manufacturers have tried to package the oils in capsules. The trouble is, there are potentially harmful side effects of these pills, especially for people on anticoagulant drugs and people with non-insulin-dependent diabetes. Also, the long-term effects of taking these pills has not yet been determined. The best advice is to stay away from fish oil pills. If you want to use fish oils to protect your heart, regularly include fish in your diet.

Which foods are high in the "good" cholesterol, HDL-cholesterol?

In a word, none. Even though the cholesterol you eat comes from many different animal sources, it's all in the same chemical form. Dietary cholesterol is absorbed into your bloodstream and goes to the liver for processing. This is where HDL- and LDL-cholesterol production and clearance take place. Many factors, including the type and amount of fat and cholesterol you eat, influence the amount of cholesterol in your blood. Your HDL level is affected by your smoking status, physical activity level, and weight loss.

Does fiber affect my blood cholesterol level?

Yes. Some studies indicate that one type of dietary fiber, soluble fiber, may help reduce blood cholesterol levels. Of course, this fiber must be eaten as part of a low-fat, low-cholesterol diet. Soluble fiber is found in oatmeal, oat bran, fruits, and legumes. It's a good idea to regularly include these foods in your diet.

I don't have high blood pressure. Do I still have to watch my sodium intake?

It's wise to limit the salt in your diet whether you have high blood pressure or not. Why? Because some people with normal blood pressure are "salt sensitive." That is, the more sodium they eat, the higher their blood pressure rises. But there's no way to determine who those people are. Since most people consume many times more sodium than the body requires, the AHA recommends that all people restrict their intake to no more than 3,000 milligrams per day.

I heard the French eat high-fat diets but because they drink a lot of red wine, they don't have as many heart attacks. I don't like wine, but I'll start drinking it if it will help protect my heart.

A news broadcast started the red wine rumor. It reported that there are more deaths from heart attack in the United States than France. It suggested that the difference may be because of red wine consumption. Unfortunately, it failed to point out that death rates from heart attack have decreased dramatically in the U.S. since 1968. In France, the death rate declined only slightly for the same period.

The news report mentioned the difference in red wine consumption between the Americans and the French, but did not address other critical issues. Was it red wine consumption that kept the French from having heart attacks? Or was it genetics, obesity, physical activity, cigarette smoking, or other lifestyle factors?

Drinking moderate amounts of alcohol (one or two drinks) has been associated with reduced risk of coronary artery disease, probably due in part to increased HDL levels. But it remains to be seen whether red wine has a different effect from other alcoholic beverages. The AHA recommends that if you don't drink now, don't start. If you do drink, limit yourself to no more than two drinks per day.

I have started to eat a clove of garlic a day to ward off heart disease (and vampires!). Am I wasting my time?

Some research indicates that it might help, but the scientific jury is still out. More studies need to be done before we know for certain whether garlic has any truly beneficial effect on heart disease. In the meantime, focus on heart disease prevention strategies that we know will work: Eat a diet low in saturated fat and cholesterol, attain a healthy weight, and don't smoke. Control your blood pressure, keep your cholesterol level below 200 mg/dl, and be physically active.

What is all the hoopla I've been hearing about antioxidants?

Some studies suggest that certain vitamins—E, C, and beta-carotene (a form of vitamin A)—have potential health-promoting properties. They seem to prevent a process called "oxidation," which causes damage to cells. The early studies are promising, but the topic needs much more study before a sweeping recommendation for supplementation can be made. The AHA recommends at least five servings per day of fruits and vegetables, which are natural sources of these vitamins, plus a good source of fiber and minerals.

Can I drink coffee and still have a healthy heart?

It looks good for coffee lovers. Studies show that caffeine may increase blood pressure slightly for a brief period after drinking coffee. But the regular ingestion of caffeine has not been associated with a greater likelihood of having high blood pressure. If you use cream in your coffee and you're a big coffee drinker, however, you could be getting a lot of extra saturated fat. A good rule to follow is

"everything in moderation." Too much of anything—even if it's good—may be harmful.

*I don't always eat right. Should I take a multi-vitamin
and mineral supplement "just to make sure" that I get all
the nutrients I need?*

Taking vitamins sounds like an easy fix, but it's
not. The truth is, scientists don't yet know all of
the nutrients in food. They also don't know the
whole story about nutrient interaction. What they
do know is this: a vitamin and mineral supplement
will not give you all the nutrients you need. That's
because your body needs more than 40 nutrients.
Most supplements, even the high-potency ones,
provide less than 20 nutrients. Where do you get
the rest? From the foods you eat. The best thing
you can do for your body is to eat a balanced,
nutritious diet with lots of variety.

*I have been on a special diet to reduce my blood choles-
terol level. I eat nothing but fruit on Mondays, Wednes-
days, and Fridays. Tuesdays and Thursdays I eat hot dogs
and salad at each meal. On the weekends, I can eat
whatever I want. What do you think?*

Sounds like you've fallen prey to someone's irre-
sponsible marketing of a fad diet. This diet is
probably costing you money. It may also affect
your health over time since it's severely lacking in
several important food groups. Remember, the
best way to reduce cholesterol level is to eat a well-
balanced diet, low in saturated fat, excess calories,
and cholesterol.

*My doctor said I should lower my blood cholesterol level.
Why should I go to the trouble? Will it really make that
much difference?*

You bet it will. Long-term studies of healthy people with high cholesterol show that for every 1 percent they reduce their blood cholesterol level, their risk of heart disease drops 2 percent. Until recently, many doctors have hesitated to prescribe cholesterol-lowering therapies because they didn't know whether it would help patients who already have heart disease or who have had a heart attack. The latest scientific evidence shows that heart attack and angina patients who reduced their blood cholesterol levels by 25 percent reduced their risk of coronary death by 42 percent. In short, anything you can do to lower your blood cholesterol to 200 mg/dl or below is well worth the effort. It will definitely help protect you from heart disease and heart attack.

HIGHLIGHTS

Eating with Your Heart in Mind

Now you know how to shop, cook, and eat for a healthy heart. Join the millions of Americans who are trimming the fat and cutting the cholesterol—for life.

CHAPTER FIVE

Keep Your Motor
Humming with
Physical Activity

Would you buy a high-performance automobile, then leave it in the garage and never drive it? Of course not. Like a high-performance car, your heart and body were designed for *movement*.

To get the most mileage out of your heart and body, you need to play, run, dance, and walk. You need to live with *vigor*, not sit in the garage and gather dust. As the old-timers say, "It's better to wear out than rust out!"

As you'll learn in this chapter, it pays to start your engine and keep your motor humming.

 ## How Much Physical Activity
Is Enough?

The good news is that you don't have to run a marathon to help keep your heart healthy. Many studies have shown that all you need is a *moderate* level of physical fitness.

129

For example, one study followed more than 10,000 men and 3,000 women from 1970 to 1985. Doctors at a leading preventive medicine center examined these subjects and gave them exercise stress tests on a treadmill. This test determined their level of fitness. During this 15-year period, 240 men and 43 women died. As the chart on the next page shows, more people who were in the low-fitness level groups died than the people in the moderate- or high-fitness level groups. This was true for both men and women and for deaths from cardiovascular disease, cancer, and all causes of death combined.

This study was significant because it showed the importance of even *moderate* levels of physical fitness. The American Heart Association cited this study, among others, when it identified "lack of physical activity" as one of the risk factors for cardiovascular disease. The other risk factors are smoking, high blood pressure, and high blood cholesterol.

More good news is that nearly everyone can achieve the level of physical fitness necessary to reduce their risk of cardiovascular disease. You don't have to be an elite athlete to be moderately fit. In fact, you don't even have to "exercise" at all.

You can get all the health benefits of being moderately fit simply by doing the following.

- Take the stairs instead of elevators;
- Park farther away from the entrance at the shopping mall;
- Get off the bus a few blocks before your actual destination; and
- Do household chores yourself instead of paying someone else to do them.

These daily tasks add up in a way that can help you improve your fitness level. You don't have to put on special exercise clothes, go to a fitness center, or

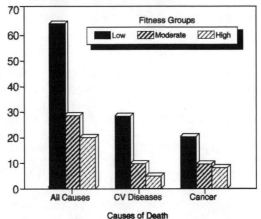

Death Rates by Fitness Groups, Men
Age-Adjusted Death Rate/10,000

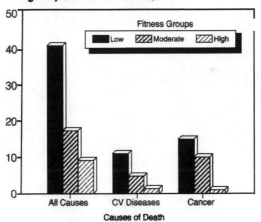

Death Rates by Fitness Groups, Women
Age-Adjusted Death Rate/10,000

FIGURE 7
Death Rates by Fitness Groups*

* Fitness Group was determined by an exercise stress test.

buy exercise equipment. You don't have to prepare a formal "exercise program." All it takes is making the decision to do something to get you moving—and *out* of the "low" fitness category.

Janet's job as an administrative assistant was sedentary until her boss was injured and confined to crutches. To accommodate the injury, the boss was moved to an empty office downstairs and around the corner from Janet's office. Over the next three months, Janet's daily physical activity increased considerably during her workday. She made frequent trips up and down the stairs to retrieve material from her boss's old office. When she repeated her fitness assessment as part of the company's worksite health promotion program, her scores were better on the cardiovascular endurance test. Janet was surprised, because she hadn't made any other changes in her daily routine. ●

Prepare to Start Your Engine

How ready are you to boost your physical activity level? Take a minute to review your answers on the Gearing Up for Change Profile on pages 35–36 as it relates to physical activity.

If you find yourself in neutral gear, look at the benefits of physical activity listed on pages 135–136. Think carefully about your reasons for becoming more active or for remaining sedentary. You may find that your reasons to become active outweigh your reasons for being inactive.

If you're in the first or second gear, you may find the information about the "lifestyle" approach to physical activity to be most beneficial to you (see pages 147–152). Adopting regular physical activity by increasing your lifestyle activity may be all you ever want to achieve. That's okay, because research shows you can get health benefits from simply increasing lifestyle-related activity.

On the other hand, if you're in the third or fourth gear, you may be interested in a traditional exercise program—or even something more vigorous! If so, we'll discuss how to start a walking or jogging program. We'll also cover injury prevention and treatment.

Get an Inspection Before You Hit the Road

Before you begin a driving vacation, it's a good idea to have your car inspected for little things that might cause you problems on the road. The same is true when you start to become more physically active.

For most people, boosting their physical activity level is a safe practice. Aside from a little muscle soreness or the odd injury, gradually increasing your physical activity level presents few problems.

But if you've always been inactive or haven't been active recently, then you need to learn the warning signs for certain problems and take a few well-advised precautions.

Most people don't need to see a doctor before they start increasing their physical activity level. That's because gradual, sensible exercise programs like the ones recommended here have minimal health risks. However, some people should seek medical advice first.

To find out if you should consult a doctor before starting or significantly increasing your physical activity, use the checklist on the next page.

If you checked one or more of the items listed, see

your doctor before you start to increase your activity level. Even if you have a problem, there's a good chance that your doctor can still design a restricted or supervised exercise program to get you started.

If you didn't check any items, feel free to start a gradual, sensible program of increased physical activity tailored to your needs.

If you feel any of the physical symptoms listed

 ## YOUR PHYSICAL ACTIVITY READINESS QUESTIONNAIRE

Mark the items that apply to you:

_____ Your doctor said you have a heart condition and recommended only medically supervised physical activity.

_____ During or right after you exercise, you frequently have pains or pressure in the left or mid-chest area, left neck, shoulder, or arm.

_____ You have developed chest pain within the last month.

_____ You tend to lose consciousness or fall over due to dizziness.

_____ You feel extremely breathless after mild exertion.

_____ Your doctor recommended you take medicine for your blood pressure or a heart condition.

_____ Your doctor said you have bone or joint problems that could be made worse by the proposed physical activity.

_____ You have a medical condition or other physical reason not mentioned here that might need special attention in an exercise program (such as insulin-dependent diabetes).

_____ You are a male over age 40 or a female over age 50, have not been physically active, and plan a relatively vigorous exercise program.

Note: This checklist has been developed from several sources, particularly the Physical Activity Readiness Questionnaire, British Columbia Ministry of Health, Department of National Health and Welfare, Canada (revised 1992).

above when you start your exercise program, contact your doctor right away. Review this list from time to time and check with your doctor if your situation changes.

Joyce is 60 years old, sedentary, and has high blood pressure. She takes a diuretic to help control her blood pressure. Like many others her age, she has aches and pains from time to time. Recently, the recreation center at her apartment began offering water aerobics, so she checked with her doctor about getting involved.

First the doctor checked her blood pressure to be sure it was under control. Then he reviewed the warning signs for heart problems and approved her participation in the water aerobics program. He was delighted that she had shown an interest in physical activity. He told Joyce that if she stayed with the aerobic activity she should lose weight. He also said she might be able to get off the blood pressure medication altogether after their next visit.

She checked back after three months and had lost six pounds. He took her off the medication and encouraged her to continue the water aerobics. After a year, she has lost a few more pounds, her blood pressure is still normal, and she's feeling great. ●

The Ten Key Benefits of Physical Activity

Increased physical activity carries the following host of benefits.

- It improves blood circulation throughout the body. The heart, lungs, and other organs and muscles work together more effectively.

- It improves your body's ability to use oxygen and provide the energy needed for movement.
- It can help reduce high blood pressure in some people. It may also help prevent high blood pressure.
- It is linked with increased HDL cholesterol levels. Remember, HDL has been called "good" cholesterol. That's because research has shown that high levels of HDL are linked with a lower risk of coronary artery disease.
- It can help smokers cut down or stop smoking.
- Along with proper diet, it can help control weight. Excess weight increases your risk of developing high blood pressure, high blood cholesterol, and diabetes. People at their desirable weight are less likely to develop diabetes. Exercise may also decrease a diabetic person's need for insulin.
- It can strengthen and tone muscles and improve your ability to perform the functions of daily living.
- It helps people handle stress, so they can do more and not tire so easily. It bolsters self-image and increases enthusiasm and optimism.
- It's good for psychological well-being because it releases tension and helps you relax and sleep well.
- It provides an easy way to share an activity with friends or family and an opportunity to meet new friends.

Are any of these benefits likely to motivate you to be active now and stay active over your lifetime? What personal benefits do you see to physical activity? List your advantages on the next page.

⟨♥⟩ WHAT PHYSICAL ACTIVITY CAN DO FOR ME	
Now	**For the Future**
•	•
•	•
•	•
•	•

Remember, physical inactivity is one of the risk factors for heart disease. Physical activity can increase the fitness of your heart and lungs, which may help protect you against heart disease—even if you have other risk factors.

 ## Roadblocks to Physical Activity

When you're trying to make changes in your lifestyle, it's important to know your mental roadblocks. If you know what's likely to be a problem, you can make plans to deal with it. Some of the most common obstacles to physical activity are discussed below.

"I don't have enough time."

Everyone has the same 24 hours a day. Making time for physical activity means that you know the benefits of physical activity and value your health. Most people make time for things they believe are important. If you're having problems in this area, try the lifestyle approach discussed later in this chapter.

Also, interview busy people who are active regularly and ask them how they do it. When you've been active for a few months, offer to help someone else who is interested in becoming active. Being a role model for others will keep you motivated to stay active.

"I'm too tired to exercise."

It might not make sense to you at first, but exercise actually counters the effects of fatigue. People who exercise regularly report feeling more energetic afterwards. They say they sleep better, too. In fact, exercise is routinely recommended for people with chronic fatigue. That's because fatigue can also be a symptom of depression and exercise relieves both of these conditions.

"I don't have a place to exercise."

If convenience is important, consider exercising at home. Try to find a place less than 10 minutes from where you live or work. Check out the shopping malls, parks, recreation centers, YWCA's or YMCA's, fitness centers, and schools to see what opportunities they offer for activity. Many won't cost anything at all.

"I have an injury or illness that limits my exercise."

Just about everyone can do some type of physical activity, regardless of age, handicap, or health status. Even people with cardiovascular disease, hypertension, diabetes, osteoporosis, and arthritis can participate in some level of exercise. If you have concerns about the safety and effectiveness of physical activity, talk with your doctor or physical therapist.

"I think exercise is boring."

It's important to make exercise interesting and fun, something you look forward to rather than dread. You'll be more likely to stick with it if it's enjoyable.

If at first you're bored, you may try diverting your attention to other things. Read a book on a treadmill, talk with your walking partner, or listen to music. Study the landscaping or architecture of the areas you pass by. Meditate or think about spiritual things, or plan a project. Think about anything that is interesting to you. Don't think too much about your body, muscles, movements, heart rate, or breathing.

Use positive self-talk to reinforce the idea that you're enjoying your activity. Say, "This is great. I'm exercising and feeling stronger. I'm sticking to my plan. I'm nearly halfway through."

"It hurts to exercise."

The statement "No pain, no gain" is a myth. Exercise shouldn't be painful. If it is, you may be doing the wrong type of exercise, or you may have started out too hard or too fast. You could be aggravating an old injury or doing weight-bearing or high-impact activity that's wrong for you. See the chart on page 140 for examples of high-impact and low-impact activities.

There's a major difference between pain that results from an injury and the muscle soreness and stiffness that's common at the beginning of an exercise program. Learn to recognize the symptoms of overuse and how to prevent and treat them on pages 199–203. If pain persists, see your doctor.

IMPACT LEVELS OF SIXTEEN POPULAR ACTIVITIES

High-Impact	Low-Impact
Jogging/running	Walking/hiking
Basketball	Cycling
Volleyball	Stationary cycling
Hopping/jumping	Swimming
Rope skipping	Rowing
Aerobic dancing	Cross-country skiing
Downhill skiing	Stepping/stair climbing
Racquet sports	Water aerobics

Are any of these barriers likely to keep you from being active now or in the future? What personal disadvantages can you identify? List them below.

 DISADVANTAGES TO ME OF PHYSICAL ACTIVITY

Now	For the Future
•	•
•	•
•	•
•	•

 ## Breaking In a New Exercise Program

Auto manufacturers always recommend that you break in a new vehicle gradually before hitting the high speeds. The same advice applies when starting a physical activity program. Your body needs time to adjust.

To plan a physical activity program that will be effective for you, try the prescriptions below.

You'll want to choose from two possible prescriptions. One is for a traditional, structured exercise program. It's for people who enjoy moderate to vigorous activity and want to become highly fit. The other prescription uses low- and moderate-level lifestyle activities rather than structured exercises. A moderate activity program can result in significant health benefits.

The more "Yes" responses you gave to these questions, the more likely you are to be successful with the traditional approach to exercise. If you answered "No" to some or most of the questions, consider the lifestyle approach to physical activity. You can always "trade in" your lifestyle approach for a more traditional or vigorous program at a later date.

THE F.I.T. PRESCRIPTION

"F' stands for Frequency—how often you perform the exercise.

"I" stands for Intensity—how hard you works while exercising.

"T" stands for Time—how many minutes you exercise at a time.

Physical Activity Profile

To help you decide which F.I.T. prescription is more likely to work for you, circle either YES or NO for each of the following statements.

YES NO   1. Have you participated in sports or vigorous activities in the past, perhaps in high school or college?

YES NO   2. Have you been physically fit in the past, and did you like the feeling?

YES NO   3. Do you have a place to exercise that is convenient?

YES NO	4.	Do you think you'd like to exercise with a partner or a group of people?
YES NO	5.	Is it easy for you to change clothes to exercise or take a shower after exercising?
YES NO	6.	Do you find the idea of getting sweaty unappealing?
YES NO	7.	When you think of vigorous exercise, do you have a positive picture in your mind?
YES NO	8.	Do you have a regular block of time (30 to 45 minutes) that you can set aside for exercise?
YES NO	9.	Are you confident that you could follow a structured exercise program?

Let's take a closer look at your responses to the Physical Activity Profile.

1. *Previous History with Exercise*. People who have had previous experience with vigorous exercise are more likely to take it up again. The problem for some, though, is that they might start off too fast and get injured or aggravate an old injury. You can't expect to perform at the same level as you did in high school—not without a lot of practice first.

2. *Feelings of Fitness*. People who have exercised for a long time often say they continue to do it because they like the way it makes them feel. Some who use the traditional approach to exercise even report a special feeling of euphoria that comes with vigorous activity. It's been called the "runner's high." What happens is this: during exercise, the body produces substances called endorphins, which are natural pain-killers.

People who use the lifestyle approach to exercise also have a feeling of fitness. There's nothing like taking a short, brisk walk to clear the cobwebs and rejuvenate yourself.

3. *A Convenient Place to Exercise.* Some people join a health club or YMCA or YWCA near their home or work. (See pages 197–199 in this section for more information about selecting a fitness center.) Others prefer to exercise in their home on a treadmill, stationary cycle, or another piece of equipment (see pages 190–195). There are also many community options for exercising. These include schools, parks, recreation centers, and shopping malls.

If not having a convenient place to exercise is a barrier for you, the lifestyle approach to physical activity easily overcomes this problem. You can find places and ways to be active almost anywhere. Look on pages 190–197 in this section for more information about creating opportunities for activity at home, at work, and at play.

4. *Social Support.* Some people enjoy having a partner or group to exercise with, or they enjoy exercising in an environment where others are exercising. They join walking groups, aerobics dance classes, water aerobics classes, etc. If you plan sports exercise such as tennis or basketball, you'll be depending on the participation of others for your exercise. That can sometimes be frustrating.

One advantage of the lifestyle approach is that you can include others in the activity if you choose, or you can go it alone. In most situations, it won't even be obvious that you're "exercising."

Whether you choose the traditional approach or lifestyle approach, social support is the key to staying active. On pages 203–206 you'll learn more skills to help you build relationships to support your physical activity goals.

5. *Managing Exercise Routines.* If you participate in a traditional exercise program, you probably will need to change into special exercise clothes. You also

may need other exercise gear (bicycle, tire pump, helmets, gloves, fins, goggles). Managing these aspects of exercise takes time and skill.

A major advantage to the lifestyle approach to activity is that you don't need to change into special exercise attire, although you certainly can if you prefer. The only gear or equipment you need in most cases is a comfortable pair of walking shoes. (See page 179 in this section for information about selecting comfortable shoes.) Not needing special clothes or gear saves money. Not having to take a shower after exercising saves time.

6. *Sweating*. If you're going to participate in vigorous activity, you're going to sweat. Some people find heavy sweating unappealing. You can learn to manage the extent to which sweating is a problem for you. Wear sweatbands on your forehead or wrists, or carry along a small workout towel if you expect to sweat heavily. The lifestyle approach, however, provides numerous opportunities to engage in low- or moderate-intensity activity without sweating.

7. *Positive Mental Images*. Most people who adopt the traditional approach to exercise have a positive mental picture of vigorous activity and of themselves as active people. If vigorous activity doesn't create a positive picture for you or you can't imagine yourself participating in vigorous activity, remember this. Vigorous activity isn't necessary to get a health benefit. You don't have to be an athlete to be active. You can choose an active lifestyle and learn to think of yourself as an active person.

8. *Time Management*. If you're going to follow the traditional F.I.T. prescription, you'll need to set aside 20 to 40 minutes for vigorous aerobic activity at least three times a week. Add the five or more minutes that you'll need to spend warming up and cooling down

before and after exercising, and the time commitment becomes even greater. If you have to drive to another location, change clothes, or take a shower after exercising, your total time commitment could easily be an hour or more.

If you're concerned that time could be a significant barrier for you on a regular basis, you might try the lifestyle approach. It doesn't take additional time, since you're doing things (household chores, gardening) you'd be doing anyway.

9. *Self-Confidence*. When you evaluate the commitments required to follow a structured exercise program, you might not feel confident that you can do it. Past experience with the traditional prescription may have colored your views. If so, consider the lifestyle approach. Almost everyone can make the commitments to a lifestyle approach to exercise.

⬤💟 The illustration on the next page shows the energy expenditure for three women during one day. The women are about the same age and size.

The solid line represents Susan, a sedentary person. The dashed line represents Linda's energy expenditure. She goes to the gym at lunch and participates in a high-intensity aerobics class. Except for this planned leisure time exercise, Linda is otherwise sedentary. The dotted line illustrates the energy expenditure for Marilu. Her job as a travel agent is relatively sedentary, but she seeks opportunities to integrate short bouts of physical activity into her daily routine. She walks to the bus stop in the morning, gets off a few blocks early, and walks the remainder of the way to her office. She climbs stairs and delivers tickets to her customers on foot. At lunch she walks a few blocks out of her way to have lunch and do a few errands. In the evening after dinner, she walks her dog in her neighborhood.

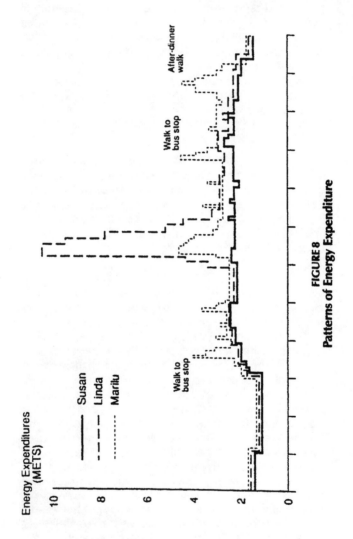

FIGURE 8
Patterns of Energy Expenditure

As you can see, leisure-time exercise and lifestyle exercise offer comparable health benefits if the total daily energy expenditure is the same. ●

Which F.I.T. Prescription Is for You?

Add up your responses to the Physical Activity Profile and determine which approach to exercise is right for you. Then follow the F.I.T. Prescription below.

F.I.T. Prescription—Lifestyle Approach

- Frequency = Be active every day or nearly every day.
- Intensity = Include moderate activity equal to brisk walking.
- Time = Be active for a minimum of 30 minutes added up over the course of a day.

F.I.T. Prescription—Traditional Approach

- Frequency = Perform aerobic exercises three to five times per week.
- Intensity = Exercise within your target heart rate zone (50 to 75 percent of your maximum heart rate).
- Time = Exercise for at least 20 to 40 minutes per session.

The Lifestyle Approach to Physical Activity

If you use the lifestyle approach, you don't have to be so structured. You simply aim to be more active in your daily life.

- Take the stairs instead of the elevator,
- Walk the dog,
- Work in the garden,
- Vacuum the carpet, and
- Rake the leaves.
- Walk or bicycle to the corner store instead of driving.
- Walk instead of using a cart when golfing.
- Mow the lawn (doesn't count if you use a riding lawn mower!),
- Do light calisthenic exercises or ride a stationary bike while you are watching the news,
- Walk and Talk—conduct one-on-one meetings at work while walking,
- Paint or wallpaper your house, and
- Bicycle or walk to work if possible.

These are ordinary activities and tasks that you can easily do in the course of a normal day. It's important to include moderate-level physical activity in your normal daily routine. Moderate intensity, equal to brisk walking (about a 15-minute mile pace), is highly recommended. One study showed that even walking at a stroller's pace (20 minutes per mile) increased cardiovascular fitness and reduced the risk of heart disease by increasing the HDL blood cholesterol (the "good" cholesterol).

THE TALK TEST. If you're participating in moderate intensity activity it's not necessary to monitor your target heart rate. Use the "Talk Test" to be sure you're not working too hard. If you're huffing and puffing so hard that you can't talk comfortably, then you're exercising too hard. If you're able to sing, you would probably benefit from picking up the pace a bit.

RATING YOUR PERCEIVED EXERTION. Another simple way to know if you're working at an appropriate level of intensity is a scale for Rating Perceived Exertion (RPE). For years, these types of scales have been used by physicians and exercise physiologists to help them communicate with their patients during exercise testing.

To use a Perceived Exertion Scale during physical activity, select the rating that best describes your sense of effort. For example, if you're feeling fairly comfortable you might assign an RPE of 2 or 3. If you're not able to talk, you would probably choose an RPE of 9 or 10. An RPE of 3 to 5 is suggested for most healthy individuals.

	PERCEIVED EXERTION SCALE
0	No perceptible change
1	Very weak
2	Weak (light)
3	Moderate
4	Somewhat strong
5	Strong
6	
7	Very strong
8	
9	
10	Very, very strong (almost maximal)
*	Maximum

The best part of the new lifestyle exercise prescription may be the "time" factor. The most common reason that people give for getting less exercise than needed is lack of time. For some people, it's next to impossible to find a significant block of time to devote to exercise on a regular basis. The new approach allows you to add up over the course of the day all of the minutes that you are engaged in moderate activity. Research has shown that you can get the same benefit from three ten-minute activity sessions as from one thirty-minute activity session of the same intensity.

THREE EASY STEPS. If it's hard for you to get started, use the following three-step process. It will help you see how easy it is to add exercise to almost any part of your day.

Step One—Two-Minute Walks. Maybe you don't think you have a 30-minute block of time to walk for exercise each day. Try to find time for several two-minute brisk walks throughout the day. Two minutes isn't really very long. Take a look at these examples.

* Go out for a two-minute walk before breakfast.
* Get off the bus a few blocks early and walk the rest of the way to work.
* Walk around your building for a break during the workday.
* Walk down the hall or upstairs to visit with a colleague instead of calling on the telephone.
* Take the stairs instead of the elevator or get off a few floors early and walk the remainder of the way.
* Walk to lunch instead of driving.
* Take a two-minute walk during lunch before returning to work.
* Park farther away at the shopping mall and walk the extra distance.
* Walk the dog in the afternoon when you get in from work.
* Take a two-minute walk with a family member after dinner.

If you could take 10 two-minute walks during the day, that would add up to 20 minutes of physical activity. List the ways you could include two-minute walks in your daily routine. Check yourself to monitor your progress. Commit to following this plan for four weeks.

I Will Do _____ Two-Minute Walks Every Day In These Ways:
•
•
•
•
•
•
•

Step Two—Five-Minute Walks. After you've been doing two-minute walks for a few weeks you'll see how easy it is to accumulate activity. Could you extend at least three of your two-minute walks to five minutes each? List at least three times that you could do five-minute walks in the space below.

I Will Do _____ Five-Minute Walks And _____ Two-Minute Walks Every Day In These Ways:
•
•
•
•
•
•
•

Don't give up the two-minute walks. Now you're up to nearly 30 minutes of physical activity a day. Try this plan for four weeks and see how you feel.

Step Three—Ten-Minute Walks. After a few weeks' experience with five-minute walks, then move to ten-minute walks. Don't give up any of the times that you walk, even the two-minute walks. List the times for your ten-minute walks in the space below.

	I Will Do _____ Ten-Minute Walks, _____ Five-Minute Walks, And _____ Two-Minute Walks Every Day In These Ways:

• _____
• _____
• _____
• _____
• _____
• _____
• _____

Can you include three ten-minute walks and several two-minute or five-minute walks over the course of the day? If so, you'll be well on your way to making physical activity a habit for life.

The Traditional Approach to Exercise

If you're opting for the traditional approach to exercise, your goal will be to improve your cardiovascular fitness. To do this, you need to monitor the intensity of your exercise by keeping track of your target heart rate zone.

TARGET HEART RATE ZONE. To determine your target heart rate zone you need to know your maximum heart rate, or the fastest your heart can beat. To find out your maximum heart rate, subtract your age from 220, which is the maximum heart rate of a baby at birth. Your maximum heart rate declines one beat per minute each year.

The target heart rate zone is between 50 and 75 percent of your maximum heart rate. Any exercise above 75 percent of your maximum heart rate may be too strenuous for you to sustain unless you are in excellent shape. Exercise below 50 percent may do little to improve your cardiovascular fitness.

As the table on page 155 shows, for a 40-year-old, the target zone is 90–135 beats per minute. A 48-year-old would choose age 50, the closest age on the chart, and see that the target zone is 85–127 beats per minute.

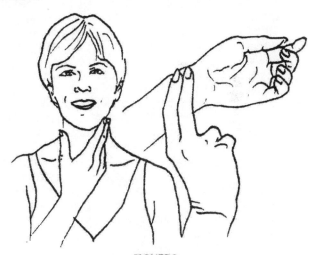

FIGURE 9
Taking the Pulse at the Neck and Wrist

TRACKING YOUR EXERCISE PULSE RATE. To see if you are within your target heart rate zone, take your pulse a third to halfway through the workout and also immediately after you stop exercising. Always keep moving while taking an exercise pulse rate.

- Place the tips of your first two fingers lightly over one of the blood vessels on your neck (carotid arteries) located to the left or right of your Adam's apple. Another convenient pulse spot is the inside of your wrist just below the base of the thumb. (See Figure 9 on page 153.)
- Count your pulse for 10 seconds and multiply by six or use the 10-second conversion chart below to obtain your number of beats per minute.
- Remember to keep moving while you're taking your pulse. If you stop too quickly, blood can pool in your legs and you may feel lightheaded.
- Practice taking your pulse until you can do it quickly. Your heart rate begins to decline rapidly when you stop exercising, so you could underestimate your target heart rate if you miss a few beats.
- If your pulse falls within your target zone, you're doing fine. If it is below your target zone, exercise a little harder next time. And if you're above your target zone, back off a little in intensity. Don't try to exercise at your maximum heart rate—that's working too hard.
- Once you know what it feels like to be exercising within your target zone, it becomes easier to exercise at the right pace. During the first three months, make sure by checking your pulse at least once each week. Continue to check it periodically after that.

	YOUR TARGET HEART RATE	
Age	Target Heart Rate Zone 50–75%	Average Maximum Heart Rate 100%
20 years	100–150 beats/min.	200
25 years	98-146 beats/min.	195
30 years	95–142 beats/min.	190
35 years	93–138 beats/min.	185
40 years	90–135 beats/min.	180
45 years	88–131 beats/min.	175
50 years	85–127 beats/min.	170
55 years	83–123 beats/min.	165
60 years	80–120 beats/min.	160
65 years	78–116 beats/min.	155
70 years	75–113 beats/min.	150

The above figures are averages and should be used as general guidelines.

Note: A few high blood pressure medicines lower the maximum heart rate and thus the target zone rate. If you are taking high blood pressure medications, call your doctor to find out if your exercise program should be adjusted.

WARMING UP (5 TO 10 MINUTES). You'll need to warm up for at least five minutes before exercising to give your body a chance to get ready for the more vigorous activity that will follow. Start at a slow to moderate pace and gradually increase it by the end of the five-minute warm-up period. If you plan to do especially vigorous activity, increase your warm-up time to nearly 10 minutes. Try to reach your target heart rate at the end of your warm-up period. Stretching is an excellent way to get your body ready for more vigorous activity. Brisk walking will get your heart rate up to the target zone.

10-SECOND PULSE RATE CONVERSION CHART

10 Second Pulse Count	Pulse Rate in Beats/Minute	10 Second Pulse Count	Pulse Rate in Beats/Minute
17	102	24	144
18	108	25	150
19	114	26	156
20	120	27	162
21	126	28	168
22	132	29	174
23	138	30	180

EXERCISING WITHIN YOUR TARGET ZONE (30 TO 60 MINUTES). Gradually increase your exercise time until you reach your goal of 30 to 60 minutes. When you get in shape, you can exercise for 30 to 60 minutes, depending on the type and intensity. For example, you will burn more calories by jogging for 20 minutes than by walking for 20 minutes. So jogging will take less time than walking to burn off the same number of calories.

Examples of how to build up to the goal of 30 to 60 minutes of walking and jogging exercise are provided on pages 184–188. The exercise patterns for both of these programs are only suggested guidelines. Listen to your body and build up less quickly if needed.

COOLING DOWN (5 MINUTES). After exercising within your target zone for an appropriate time, start to slow down gradually, lowering the intensity. For example, if you're swimming, swim more slowly or change to a more leisurely stroke. If you're jogging, slow to a walk.

The cool-down period is necessary to allow your heart rate and blood pressure to return to normal. If you're exercising vigorously and stop too quickly, you could become light-headed or dizzy. The safe practice is to keep moving while cooling down gradually.

The cool-down period is an excellent time to do your flexibility exercises because your muscles are warm and your joints are limber. Stretches will be easier to do, and you may be able to extend your normal range of motion.

 ## Hitting on All Cylinders— Balanced Fitness

A car doesn't run its best if all cylinders aren't operating. Your body is the same way. It needs all three components of fitness—aerobics, flexibility, and strength—for optimal health.

Coordination, balance, agility, speed, power, and reaction time are also components of fitness. These factors are related to efficiency of movement and athletic performance rather than health. Achieving balanced fitness means that you are including all three types of activities in your lifestyle.

Aerobic activities use large muscles and challenge the circulatory system. These activities are rhythmic and repetitive. They also significantly increase the blood flow to the working muscles. To achieve cardiovascular fitness, you need to participate in aerobic activities. When your cardiovascular system is fit, you can be active for long periods of time without getting too tired. Aerobic activity also can help you achieve and maintain a healthful body weight.

Two other aspects of fitness are important: flexibility and strength. Two components of strength are muscle strength and endurance.

Flexibility is the ability to move a part of the body through its full range of motion. Stretching exercises can improve your flexibility.

Muscle strength is the maximum force that can be generated by a muscle or muscle group. People who have strong muscles can lift heavy objects, jump, pull, carry, and do other activities more easily. Strong muscles, particularly in the back and abdomen, promote good posture and help relieve low back pain. Muscle endurance is the ability of the muscles to make repeated contractions with a less than maximum load. If you can lift a weight or object many times before becoming tired, you have good muscle endurance.

AEROBIC ACTIVITY. To be sure that an activity qualifies as aerobic, you should be able to answer "yes" to all three of the following questions.

- Does it use the large muscle groups of your body, such as buttocks, thighs, and back?
- Does it increase your heart rate, and can you continue the activity for more than a few minutes?
- Does it cause you to feel warm, perspire, and breathe heavily without being really out of breath and without feeling any burning sensation in the muscles?

The chart below shows three groups of activities organized by how they affect your heart.

The activities in Group A are most vigorous and, if done regularly at a sustained level, promote a high level of fitness. Group B activities are moderately vigorous but are still excellent choices for fitness and health benefits. Group C lists low-intensity activities. Even though they are low-intensity, they still have health benefits. They can help lower your risk of heart disease if done daily.

	HEART-AT-WORK ACTIVITIES	
Group A Vigorous (High Intensity) Activities	**Group B** Moderate Activities	**Group C** Low-Intensity Activities
Aerobic dancing	Walking briskly	Badminton
Bicycling	Downhill skiing	Baseball
Cross-country skiing	Baskeball	Bowling
Hiking (uphill)	Field hockey	Croquet
Ice hockey	Football	Gardening
Jogging	Calisthenics	Golf (on foot or by cart)
Jumping rope	Handball	Housework
Rowing	Racquetball	Ping-pong
Running in place	Squash	Shuffleboard
Soccer	Tennis (singles)	Social dancing
Stair-climbing	Volleyball	Softball
Stationary cycling		Walking leisurely
Swimming		

FLEXIBILITY ACTIVITY. Stretching or flexibility exercises are often the most neglected part of a balanced fitness program. Poor flexibility can be caused by bone and joint diseases. It can also be caused by tight muscles, ligaments, and tendons—all of which can be addressed with appropriate stretching exercises. (See Figure 10 on pages 162–163.) Young people are naturally more flexible. As you age, you lose flexibility in your joints if you don't perform stretches to maintain it. Having good flexibility reduces the likelihood of injury to muscles, ligaments, and tendons. Flexibility also makes it easier to perform daily tasks and activities.

Stretching doesn't have to take a lot of time. You can stop and stretch:

- in the morning before starting the day,
- at work to relieve stress,
- before an aerobic or strength-building activity to warm-up your muscles,
- after sitting or standing for a long period of time, or
- anytime that you feel stiff.

Irving, a retired engineer and grandfather, visited his doctor for his annual checkup and fitness evaluation. He reported that overall he was feeling great: running three miles every morning, eating well, spending a lot of time with his grandchildren, and going fishing in Canada every summer. In all, life was great. Unfortunately, he said, his golf game was beginning to suffer because of stiffness in his shoulders and upper back.

He mentioned his mother's arthritis, wondering if there was a connection. Upon examining Irving's back, his doctor discovered the problem wasn't arthritis at all. The stiffness in his back was caused simply by lack of use and poor muscle tone. His doctor taught him a variety of stretching exercises to increase flexibility in his upper back. The following year Irving visited the clinic for his annual checkup. When asked about the stiffness, Irving reported he'd added 20 yards to his drive! ●

It's important to do your stretches properly or you won't get much benefit from them. There's also some risk of injury. Stretching exercises should be performed slowly and with full control. This means:

- Don't hold your breath while stretching. Maintain an even breathing rate. Inhale before the stretch and exhale during the active phase of the stretch.
- If balance is a problem, be sure that a support is nearby (a wall, chair, another person).
- Do not bounce. Bouncing does not stretch the muscles, but it could tear them.
- Don't stretch too far. Stretch just to the point where you feel mild tension in the muscle. Trying to stretch too far can cause injuries.
- Hold each stretch for 10 to 20 seconds. Perform each stretch three to five times.

Neck Stretches. While sitting or standing with your head in its normal upright position, slowly tilt your head to the left until you feel tension on the right side of your neck. Hold for 10 to 15 seconds, then return your head to the upright position. Repeat to the right side, and then toward the front. Always return to the upright position before moving on. Do not tilt the head back.

Shoulder Circles. Rotate the shoulders in the backward direction. Be sure to go through the full range of motion. Because most people have a slight case of rounded shoulders due to desk work, housework, or other tasks, forward shoulder circles aren't necessary.

Chest Stretches. Clasp your hands behind your back and stretch your chest muscles by pulling your shoulder blades together. Also, perform the chest stretch while bending forward at the waist and lifting your clasped hands away from your lower back toward the ceiling.

Upper Back Stretches. Stand with your feet shoulder-width apart and your knees slightly bent. Raise your arms out in front of you until they are level with

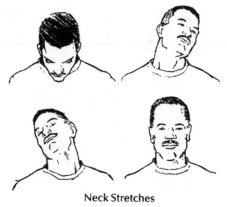

Neck Stretches

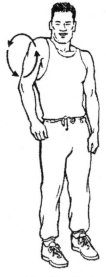

Shoulder Circles

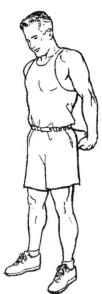

Chest Stretches

FIGURE 10
Stretching or Flexibility Activities

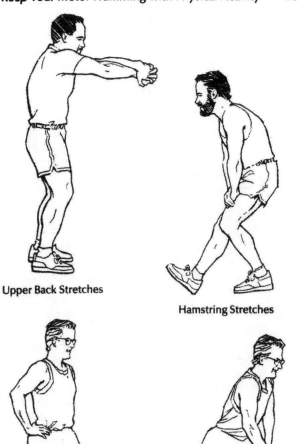

Upper Back Stretches

Hamstring Stretches

Calf Stretches

your chest. Cross your left forearm over the right and turn your palms to face each other. Lock fingers. Drop your chin to your chest, tighten your abdomen and round your back. As your arms stretch forward and your torso leans back a little, feel the shoulder blades separate from each other. Hold. Repeat, crossing your right arm over the left.

Side Bends. Stand with feet shoulder width apart. Extend one arm overhead and place the hand of the other arm on the hip. Bend to the side opposite the lifted arm. Extend the other arm overhead and repeat to the opposite side.

Thigh Stretches. Stand facing a wall. Place your right hand against the wall at shoulder level for balance. Bend your left leg at the knee. Using your left hand, grasp the top of your left foot behind you. Gently pull your heel toward your buttocks. Repeat for the other side.

Hamstring Stretches. Stand with your feet shoulder width apart and extend one foot in front of the other in a parallel position. Bend your supporting leg and keep your front leg straight, with the foot flexed. Flex your foot as much as possible to achieve the maximum stretch. Keep your weight centered between your feet. Place both hands on your thigh for upper body support.

Calf Stretches. Stand with your feet together and parallel. Step with one foot forward so that your feet are approximately one to two feet apart. Gently shift your weight onto your front leg, being sure to keep your back leg straight and your back toes directed forward. Keep both heels on the floor. You can rest your hands on your front leg for stability.

STRENGTH-BUILDING ACTIVITY—GOLD MEDAL ADVICE.
Everybody needs strength. Good muscle strength and
endurance may be the most important part of physical
fitness in the later years. Think about what you want
to be able to do when you're in your eighties or
nineties (and there's a good chance you'll live that
long). The activities of daily living, such as taking a
shower, getting dressed, or feeding yourself require a
good level of strength. Any difficulty you have now
performing these necessary tasks can eventually lead
to the need for assistance and can limit the opportunity to live independently. So build your strength now
as an investment that will pay off when you're older.

When you're young, the amount of strength you
need is determined mostly by your job and recreational pursuits. Some people, such as firefighters,
need strong muscles to lift, carry, and pull objects or
equipment as part of their job. Even if your job is
sedentary, you may enjoy leisure activities that require good muscle strength. Whether you play tennis
or golf, or enjoy digging in the garden as a hobby, you
will perform better if you have good muscle strength.

There are other benefits of building muscle
strength. Muscle (lean) tissue is more active than fat
tissue, so increasing the amount of lean tissue in your
body means your metabolic rate will increase. (Your
metabolic rate is the amount of calories you burn at
rest.) So it's easy to see why having an adequate
amount of muscle can help you achieve and maintain
a healthy weight. And strong muscles help you stand
erect with good posture. Firm and toned muscles can
enhance your appearance as well as your health.

How much exercise is needed to achieve and maintain an adequate level of strength? Many organizations
recommend that healthy adults perform a minimum of
eight to ten exercises involving the major muscle

groups a minimum of two times per week to achieve adequate strength. You should perform at least one set of eight to twelve repetitions to near fatigue for each exercise. The last few repetitions should be difficult to do. Allow a brief period of rest between sets for muscles to recover.

You can build strength in several ways. Calisthenic exercises use the body's weight and the force of gravity as resistance. An advantage of calisthenics is that no equipment is needed. For some muscle groups, such as the ones in your abdomen, calisthenics may be the exercise of choice.

Handheld weights, rubber resistance bands, and weight machines are other options for strength-building exercises. An advantage of weight equipment over calisthenics is your ability to adjust the resistance more easily as you get stronger.

Your body doesn't know what type of resistance you're using. It's not the equipment that produces the results; it's how you use it. All four types of resistance exercises can be effective in helping you improve your muscle strength and endurance. Lifestyle, vocational, and recreational activities such as gardening, carpentry work, and gymnastics can also help build strength.

Take time to learn to do strength-building exercises properly. Proper technique is safer and more efficient. And, you'll progress faster. (See Figure 11 on pages 168–169.) Here are tips to help you get started.

- Do a few stretches to warm up the muscles before applying resistance. Move the joints through the same range of motion that you'll do when you add resistance.
- Begin with exercises that work the large muscle groups (shoulders, back, chest, thighs) before proceeding to the smaller, individual muscles (arms, calves).

- Alternate exercises requiring a "push" motion with those requiring a "pull" motion.
- Work the joint through the full range of motion to build strength and increase flexibility.
- Maintain control (don't jerk), and go all the way from fully stretched to fully contracted.
- Take your time. Stress the muscle slowly and gradually.
- Breathe properly. Don't hold your breath or grunt. Exhale as the force is applied.
- Stretch at the end of exercise session to cool down. Stretching will be easier than at the beginning because the muscles are warm.
- If you're using weight machines or free weights, check your equipment regularly to ensure that weights are secure.
- Wear rubber-soled shoes for secure footing. Wear clothing that allows for the evaporation of perspiration.
- Drink plenty of water before and during physical activity, particularly in hot or humid conditions.
- Allow at least 48 hours of rest between strength training workouts involving a specific muscle group. Muscles need time to recover when they have been completely fatigued.

Push-Ups (Shoulders, Chest, Arms). With your toes on the ground, lean forward and put your hands on the ground about shoulder width apart. Keeping your back straight, lower your upper body to the ground and back up again. Inhale while lowering your body; exhale while raising your body.

Modified Push-Ups. Same as above, except do these with your knees instead of your toes on the ground. Keep your back straight. Inhale while lowering body; exhale while raising body.

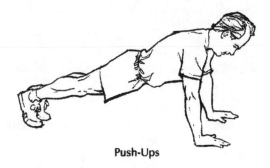

Push-Ups

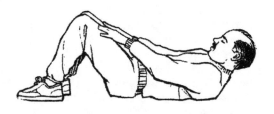

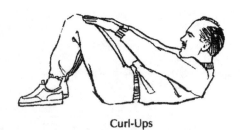

Curl-Ups

FIGURE 11
Calisthentics for Building Strength

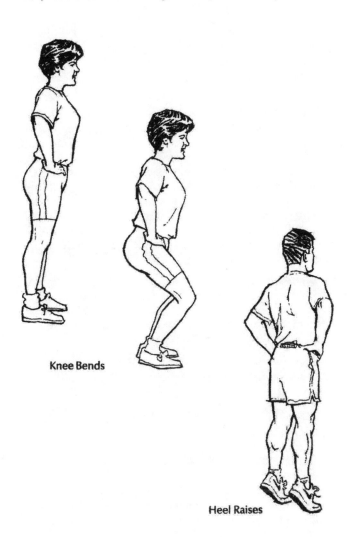

Knee Bends

Heel Raises

Curl Ups (Abdominals). Begin in a horizontal position with knees bent at a 70–90 degree angle and the palms of your hands resting on your thighs. Lift your shoulders off the ground and slide your fingers up toward your knees. Return to starting position and repeat.

Chair Dips (Shoulders, Upper Back, Arms). Find a chair or bench that will stay firmly in place. Stand with your back to the chair, as if you were going to sit on it. Slowly bend your knees and reach behind you until you can grasp the front edge of the seat with both hands. Transfer your weight to your hands and slowly slide your feet out in front of you. Keep your feet shoulder width apart and your knees bent. Lower yourself and then push yourself up by straightening your elbows. Exhale when pushing up; inhale when lowering your body.

Knee Bends (Thighs). Place your feet shoulder distance apart, toes pointed straight ahead, and hands on your hips. Squat until your thighs are parallel to the ground. Keep your back straight. Inhale while squatting; exhale while straightening your legs.

Heel Raises (Calves). Standing erect with your hands on your hips, rise up on your toes as high as possible. Return to starting position. Place a 1- to 2-inch-thick block of wood or book under your toes for a more challenging heel raise. Exhale while rising up on toes; inhale on the return.

ACHIEVING BALANCED FITNESS

Joe is thirty-eight years old and works as a computer software salesman. He played football in college. Except for an old knee injury that bothers him from time to time, he thinks he's in good health. His exercise program consists of heavy weightlifting five days a week.

Sue, a forty-seven-year-old mother of three, teaches physical education at an elementary school. She hasn't missed work due to illness during the last year. Running is her favorite exercise. Her training program consists of running 35 to 40 miles per week. She plans to run her first marathon this year.

Jerry is fifty-six years old and a lawyer by profession. He had bypass surgery when he was fifty-two and it changed his life. Now he walks briskly for 30 to 45 minutes five days a week. He also spends 30 minutes three days per week working out with light dumbbells at home. To relieve stress, he's taken up gardening and works in the yard at least four hours every week.

Which person has the more balanced fitness program?

Although it's less vigorous than Joe's (the weight-lifter) or Sue's (the marathon runner), Jerry's fitness program is more balanced. His exercises include activities to develop cardiovascular endurance, flexibility, muscle strength, and endurance. ●

Cross-training can help you achieve balanced fitness and overcome at least two of the most common

CROSS-TRAINING PLAN	
Day	**Activity**
Monday & Friday	Stretching, Walking, Calisthenics
Tuesday & Thursday	Stretching, Weight Training, Stationary Cycling
Wednesday	Stretching, Tennis
Weekends	Stretching, Recreation, Gardening

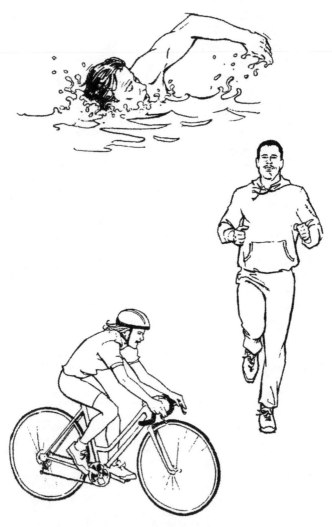

FIGURE 12
Popular Sports Activities

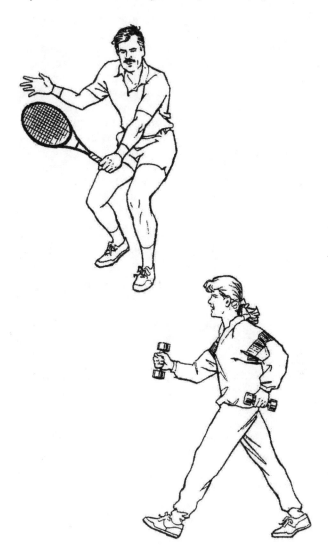

barriers to exercise or physical activity: boredom and lack of results. By including a variety of exercises and activities, cross-training keeps you challenged and motivated to stay with your program. (See Figure 12 on pages 172–173.) And because you're changing activities frequently, you're not overusing the same muscles. Plus, you're less likely to get injured.

Use the following Exercise Planner to develop a cross-training plan. It will help you to have an idea of what you intend to do for the week in advance. You can combine different types of exercise or change the sequence of the same exercises. There's also space for you to record a few measurements.

EXERCISE PLANNER
Week of: _____

Day	Time	Activity	Place
Monday _____
Preparations/reminders: _____
Tuesday _____
Preparations/reminders: _____
Wednesday _____
Preparations/reminders: _____
Thursday _____
Preparations/reminders: _____
Friday _____
Preparations/reminders: _____
Saturday _____
Preparations/reminders: _____
Sunday _____
Preparations/reminders: _____

Date _____ Weight _____ Resting Heart Rate_____

The One-Mile Fitness Test

Before you get started on a physical activity program, it's a good idea to get a general idea of your current fitness level. Here's an easy, do-it-yourself fitness test that you can use now. If you're taking blood pressure medicine, heart or lung medicine, antidepressants, drugs to help you lose weight, or any drug that depresses or increases your heart rate, this test may not be valid for you.

PRECAUTIONS. Review the Physical Activity Readiness Questionnaire on page 134 before you perform this fitness test. If there has been a change in your health since your last doctor visit, you may want to check again to be sure it's safe for you to perform this test.

- If you experience any unusual pain or discomfort during any part of the test, STOP IMMEDI-ATELY and consult your doctor.

PREPARING FOR THE TEST

- Avoid caffeinated beverages (coffee, tea, colas) or a heavy meal for at least three hours before the test.
- Find a measured, one-mile track at a school, park, or recreation center. If you want to measure your own course, find a smooth, level surface.
- Bring a stopwatch or a watch with a second hand, a pencil and paper, and wear comfortable clothing and walking shoes.
- Don't perform the test outdoors on days that are extremely hot or cold and windy.
- Learn to take your pulse and practice before taking this test.

- Walk or stretch for several minutes before starting the test.

TAKING THE TEST. Start walking as quickly as you can to get your heart rate up to at least 110 beats per minute without straining. To check your heart rate at your neck or wrist, count the number of pulse beats in six seconds and add a zero. (This will give you the beats per minute.) For example, if you count 12 beats in six seconds, your heart rate is 120 beats per minute.

Measure your pulse five minutes into your walk. Make sure your pulse remains above 110 beats per minute. Maintain a constant pace as you walk. Remember to keep your breathing smooth and regular.

Record the time (in minutes and seconds) that it took you to walk one mile. Most people take between 10 and 20 minutes to walk a mile. When you finish walking the mile, keep moving slowing, and immediately take your pulse. Write this number down, too. Continue to walk slowly for a few minutes to allow your heart rate and blood pressure to return to normal levels.

ONE-MILE FITNESS TEST

MY TIME ____ min. ____ sec.

WEIGHT____

AGE____

DATE

MY FINAL PULSE _____

                             beats/minute

FITNESS LEVEL

____ Low

____ Moderate

____ High

SCORING YOUR TEST. Find the Chart for Scoring the One-Mile Fitness Test for your sex on pages 376–379 in Appendix A. Find your age range and your heart rate. If your exact pulse isn't shown, round it off to the nearest 10 beats.

To the right of that, you'll see the one-mile walk times for low, medium, and high fitness levels. You may need to add or subtract time to your score if your weight differs from the amount shown on the chart. That's because for every ten pounds of extra weight, you must walk 15 seconds faster to qualify for a given fitness category. To figure that, add 15 seconds to your overall time for every 10 pounds over the weight shown as about average. On the other hand, for every 10 pounds under the average weight listed, you can walk 15 seconds slower and still qualify for a fitness category. To figure your score, subtract 15 seconds from your total time for every 10 pounds you are under the listed average.

EXAMPLES

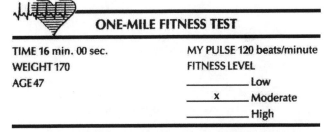

ONE-MILE FITNESS TEST

TIME 16 min. 00 sec.　　　　MY PULSE 120 beats/minute
WEIGHT 170　　　　　　　　FITNESS LEVEL
AGE 47　　　　　　　　　　＿＿＿＿＿＿ Low
　　　　　　　　　　　　　＿＿＿x＿＿ Moderate
　　　　　　　　　　　　　＿＿＿＿＿＿ High

If, for example, you were a 47-year-old man who weighed 170 pounds and walked the one-mile course with a heart rate of 120 in 16 minutes, you would be at the moderate fitness level. Because your weight is within five pounds of the average shown, you wouldn't have to add or subtract time to your score.

ONE-MILE FITNESS TEST

MY TIME 17 min. 30 sec.	MY PULSE 150 beats/minute
WEIGHT 145	FITNESS LEVEL
AGE 33	_____x_____ Low
*Add 30 seconds	_____ Moderate
	_____ High

If you were a 33-year-old woman who weighed 145 pounds and walked the course with a heart rate of 150 in 17 minutes 30 seconds, you would be at a low fitness level. That's because, at 20 pounds over the 125 norm, you must add 30 seconds to your overall time for a total of 18 minutes.

Of course, this test is just a rough estimate of your actual fitness. But it *is* a place to start. After about eight weeks of regular physical activity, test yourself again to check your progress. Over time, you'll find you can cover the mile faster or your heart rate will be lower.

First Gear— Starting a Customized Exercise Program

Walking has become a popular mode of activity, and rightly so. There are numerous advantages. Here are nine:

- It's part of your daily routine. It doesn't have to take time away from other activities. You can walk to work, walk to lunch, walk while shopping at the mall, or walk for sightseeing on vacation.
- It's inexpensive to do. All you really need is a good pair of walking shoes.

- It's easy to do. You don't have to learn any new skills (although instruction in some of the more advanced techniques could be helpful).
- It's convenient. You can walk almost any place and time, and in all but the most severe weather.
- It's easy to stick with a walking program. The dropout rate for walking is less than for other exercise programs.
- It's safe. The impact is only a fraction of that of jogging or some aerobic dancing. You're not likely to get injured when walking.
- It's effective, especially if you're trying to control your weight. Because it's easy to do, you can walk longer and burn more calories.
- It's weight bearing, so it helps make your bones stronger.
- It's fun. You can do it alone, with a partner, or a pet.

Whether you've chosen a traditional exercise program or the lifestyle approach, walking can meet your needs. You can walk for a period of time all or once (30 to 60 minutes) or add up the duration of shorter walks over the course of the day. What counts is the total amount of physical activity you do. It all adds up to good health.

7 KEY POINTS FOR SELECTING WALKING SHOES. Choose a shoe designed especially for walking or hiking. Casual shoes and sneakers are less suited for the movement of walking and could cause problems because they don't provide enough cushioning and support. Wear thick socks when you try on walking shoes at the store and look for shoes with these features:

- Lightweight;
- Thick soles of rubber or crepe that will cushion the foot;

- Firm support behind the heel to prevent sliding;
- A slightly elevated heel;
- Arch support;
- Strong leather or fabric uppers, to let your foot breathe; and
- A good fit. (Make sure you have enough room around and above the toe and about 1/4 inch between the longest toe and the front of the shoe.)

FOCUS ON FEELING GOOD. As you're implementing your walking program, consider how you're feeling—physically and emotionally.

- Does walking make you feel better?
- Do you feel more relaxed and less tense after walking?
- Does walking help to clear your mind?
- Are you beginning to picture yourself as an active person?
- Is walking helping you manage your weight?
- Are you feeling stronger?
- Are you feeling less tired?
- Are you sleeping better?
- Is it getting easier to climb stairs and do certain chores?
- Are you feeling more confident?
- Is your pulse rate decreasing?
- Is walking becoming a habit for you?
- Do you miss your walks if you don't do them?

 A Traditional Walking Program

You've been walking since you were two years old, so no real instructions are needed. These tips may help you, though, if you want to start a traditional fitness walking program. Review the F.I.T. prescription, page 141, and look at the suggested walking program on the next page.

WALKING TIPS. If you're not active now, you'll want to begin slowly with a 10- to 15-minute walk three times a week. As you become more fit, you can do longer sessions.

If you're already active, try for a minimum of 30 minutes at your target heart rate zone. Walk at least three or four times per week (every other day). To experience the full cardiovascular benefits and make steady progress, you'll want to walk at least three times a week.

YOUR WALKING GOALS. How much walking do you need to do to reach a moderate level of fitness in your walking program? How much for a high level? It's simple. Follow the fitness goals below.

Moderate Fitness.

Women: Walk two miles in less than 30 minutes at least three days per week, or walk two miles in 30 to 40 minutes five to six times per week.

Men: Walk two miles in less than 27 minutes at least three days per week, or walk two miles in 30 to 40 minutes six to seven times per week.

High Fitness.

Women: Walk two miles in less than 30 minutes five or six days per week.

Men: Walk two and a half miles in less than 37.5 minutes six to seven days per week.

Younger people probably need to do a bit more, and older people could do a bit less than these examples.

---

9 TIPS FOR FITNESS WALKING

- Warm up by performing a few stretches. See pages 162–163 for illustrations.

- Think tall as you walk. Stand straight with your head level and your shoulders relaxed.

- Your heel will hit the surface first. Use smooth movements rolling from heel to toe.

- Keep your hands free and let your arms swing naturally at your sides in opposition to your legs.

- When you're ready to pick up the pace, quicken your step and lengthen your stride. But don't compromise your upright posture or smooth, comfortable movements.

- To increase your intensity, burn more calories, and tone your upper body, bend your arms at the elbows and pump your arms. Keep your elbows close to your body.

- Breathe in and out naturally, rhythmically, and deeply.

- Use the "Talk Test" (page 148) to check your intensity, or take your pulse to see if you are within your target zone (page 153).

- Cool down during the last three to five minutes by gradually slowing your pace to a stroll.

CLOTHING FOR BEING ACTIVE. Unless you're exercising indoors, the weather will most likely determine the clothing you wear to walk.

Summer. Wear cool, loose, lightweight clothing so that your body heat can escape.

- Add a hat, visor, and sunglasses.
- Protect your skin with sunscreen.
- Walk in early morning or evening.

- Drink water before you start, and carry some with you if you'll be out for more than a half hour.

Winter. Wear clothing in layers to retain your body heat. You can remove or open outer layers if you get too warm.

- Add a nylon windbreaker if wind chill is a factor.
- Try to stay dry. If your clothing becomes wet, try to change as quickly as possible.
- Add a wool cap and mittens. Layering clothing on your hands and feet can also help you stay warm.

IMPORTANT SAFETY PRECAUTIONS.

- Medical Clearance—Review the Physical Activity Readiness Questionnaire on page 134 to be sure that it's safe for you to participate in a walking program.
- After Dark—If you're walking after dark, wear bright-colored clothing or reflective markers.
- Sickness—Don't walk or exercise if you have a fever. Wait at least 24 hours before you start exercising again.
- Warning Signs—Know the signs and symptoms of heart attack (see page xviii), and stroke (see page xviii).
- Route—Avoid unpopulated areas, deserted streets, overgrown trails, poorly lighted areas, parked cars, and bushes. Watch for dogs. Vary your route from time to time.
- Personal Safety—If you're walking alone, tell someone your route and when you'll return. Don't take a large amount of money or wear expensive jewelry. Strap on a lightweight pack for items such as keys, identification, and a small amount of money.

- Traffic—Always face the traffic and watch out for cars and bicycles. If you wear a headset, keep the volume low enough to be able to hear the sounds of traffic.
- Pollution/Air Quality—Don't exercise outdoors if the air quality is poor due to industrial pollution, ozone, pollen, or mold.
- Altitude—Slow your pace if you're walking at higher altitudes than you're accustomed to.

Shifting Gears—A Sample Walking and Jogging Program

Now that you know the rules of the road, here's a sample walking program to get you started. Following this is a sample jogging program for those who want more vigorous exercise. If you're over forty and haven't been active, don't begin with a program as strenuous as jogging. Instead, allow yourself to become thoroughly comfortable with the walking program and then shift gears into the third week of the jogging program.

A SAMPLE WALKING PROGRAM

	Target Zone			
	Warm Up	Exercising	Cool Down	Total Time
Week 1*	Walk 5 min.	Walk briskly 5 min.	Walk more slowly 5 min.	15 min.
Week 2	Walk 5 min.	Walk briskly 7 min.	Walk more slowly 5 min.	17 min.
Week 3	Walk 5 min.	Walk briskly 9 min.	Walk more slowly 5 min.	19 min.

| | Target Zone | | | |
	Warm Up	Exercising	Cool Down	Total Time
Week 4	Walk 5 min.	Walk briskly 11 min.	Walk more slowly 5 min.	21 min.
Week 5	Walk 5 min.	Walk briskly 13 min.	Walk more slowly 5 min.	23 min.
Week 6	Walk 5 min.	Walk briskly 15 min.	Walk more slowly 5 min.	25 min.
Week 7	Walk 5 min.	Walk briskly 18 min.	Walk more slowly 5 min.	28 min.
Week 8	Walk 5 min.	Walk briskly 20 min.	Walk more slowly 5 min.	30 min.
Week 9	Walk 5 min.	Walk briskly 23 min.	Walk more slowly 5 min.	33 min.
Week 10	Walk 5 min.	Walk briskly 26 min.	Walk more slowly 5 min.	36 min.
Week 11	Walk 5 min.	Walk briskly 28 min.	Walk more slowly 5 min.	38 min.
Week 12	Walk 5 min.	Walk briskly 30 min.	Walk more slowly 5 min.	40 min.

*Do one exercise session at least three times a week during each week of the program.

From Week 13 on: Check your pulse periodically to see if you are exercising within your target zone. As you become more fit, try exercising within the upper range of your target zone. Gradually increase your brisk walking time to 30 to 60 minutes, three or four times a week. Remember that while your goal is to build your cardiovascular fitness, you also want to have fun!

A SAMPLE HEART-SMART JOGGING PROGRÀM

	Target Zone			
	Warm Up	**Exercising**	**Cool Down**	**Total Time**
Week 1*	Walk 5 min.; then stretch and limber up.	Walk 10 min.; try not to stop.	Walk 3 min. more slowly; stretch 2 min.	20 min.
Week 2	Walk 5 min.; then stretch and limber up.	Walk 5 min.; jog 1 min.; walk 5 min.; jog 1 min.	Walk 3 min.; stretch 2 min.	22 min.
Week 3	Walk 5 min.; then stretch and limber up.	Walk 5 min.; jog 3 min.; walk 5 min.; jog 3 min.	Walk 3 min.; stretch 2 min.	26 min.
Week 4	Walk 5 min.; then stretch and limber up.	Walk 4 min.; jog 5 min.; walk 4 min.; jog 5 min.	Walk 3 min.; stretch 2 min.	28 min.
Week 5	Walk 5 min.; then stretch and limber up.	Walk 4 min.; jog 5 min.; walk 4 min.; jog 5 min.	Walk 3 min.; stretch 2 min.	28 min.
Week 6	Walk 5 min.; then stretch and limber up.	Walk 4 min.; jog 6 min.; walk 4 min.; jog 6 min.	Walk 3 min.; stretch 2 min.	30 min.

	Target Zone			
	Warm Up	**Exercising**	**Cool Down**	**Total Time**
Week 7	Walk 5 min.; then stretch and limber up.	Walk 4 min.; jog 7 min.; walk 4 min.; jog 7 min.	Walk 3 min.; stretch 2 min.	32 min.
Week 8	Walk 5 min.; then stretch and limber up.	Walk 4 min.; jog 8 min.; walk 4 min.; jog 8 min.	Walk 3 min.; stretch 2 min.	34 min.
Week 9	Walk 5 min.; then stretch and limber up.	Walk 4 min.; jog 9 min.; walk 4 min.; jog 9 min.	Walk 3 min.; stretch 2 min.	36 min.
Week 10	Walk 5 min.; then stretch and limber up.	Walk 4 min.; jog 13 min.	Walk 3 min.; stretch 2 min.	27 min.
Week 11	Walk 5 min.; then stretch and limber up.	Walk 4 min.; jog 15 min.	Walk 3 min.; stretch 2 min.	29 min.
Week 12	Walk 5 min.; then stretch and limber up.	Walk 4 min.; jog 17 min.	Walk 3 min.; stretch 2 min.	31 min.

(continued)

| | Target Zone | | | |
	Warm Up	Exercising	Cool Down	Total Time
Week 13	Walk 5 min.; then stretch and limber up.	Walk 2 min.; jog slowly 2 min.; jog 17 min.	Walk 3 min.; stretch 2 min.	31 min.
Week 14	Walk 5 min.; then stretch and limber up.	Walk 1 min.; jog slowly 3 min.; jog 17 min.	Walk 3 min.; stretch 2 min.	31 min.
Week 15	Walk 5 min.; then stretch and limber up.	Slowly jog 3 min.; jog 17 min.	Walk 3 min.; stretch 2 min.	30 min.

*Do an exercise session at least three times a week during each week of the program.

From Week 16 on: Check your pulse periodically to see if you are exercising within your target zone. As you become more fit, try exercising within the upper range of your target zone. Gradually increase your jogging tiime from 20 to 30 minutes (or more, up to 60 minutes), three or four times a week. Remember that while your goal is to attain cardiovascular fitness, try to work in some fun!

Advanced Walking Techniques

After you've mastered a standard walking program, you may be ready for some advanced techniques. The following techniques are guaranteed to give your walking program some additional challenge.

WALKING WITH HAND WEIGHTS. This walking technique can raise the heart rate and burn more calories for an even greater fitness benefit. But this technique is not for everyone. If you have heart disease, high blood pressure, or any musculoskeletal problems (strains, tendonitis, bursitis, etc.), don't add weights of any kind when walking. Never use ankle weights. They can increase your risk of injury.

Begin with small hand or wrist weights—one-half or one pound in each hand. Increase your weight load gradually in one-half pound increments. Don't go beyond three pounds per hand.

Warm up a few minutes longer when walking with hand weights. Grip the weights gently and move your arms within the natural range of motion. Be sure to maintain proper posture and walking form when walking with weights.

RACEWALKING—PICKING UP THE PACE. If you've seen racewalkers, it's pretty impressive what they can do. Some move at a pace nearly as fast as runners, six to nine miles per hour. The difference between racewalking and jogging/running is that race walking requires that you keep one foot on the ground at all times. At about a 12-minute mile pace, it becomes easier and more efficient to run than to walk. Therefore, walking burns more calories than running at a 12-minute-mile or faster pace.

Racewalking provides an excellent fitness benefit and challenge. However, there is an increased risk of injury due to the vigorous hip movements. If you're interested in this type of walking, find an instructor who can teach you proper form.

UPHILL WALKING. Climbing stairs and hiking uphill are excellent ways to increase the intensity of walking. If hilly terrain is not available to you, a stair-climbing machine or treadmill can provide a consistent pace against gravity.

Getting a Jump Start on Fitness: Creating Opportunities to Be Active

The following pages will help you learn ways to integrate physical activity into your daily life to get you on the road to fitness.

NO MORE EXCUSES

Physical Inactivity Cues	Possible Solutions
• Maid for light housekeeping	• Do the work yourself
• Power law mower	• Get a standard lawn mover
• Vaccum	• Work faster to increase intensity
• Car for short errands	• Ride a bicycle
• Golf cart	• Walk instead
• Putting dog in backyard	• Taking dog on a walk
Exercise Equipment	
• Broken	• Get equipment repaired
• Stored out of sight	• Make it visible
• Exercise clothing	• Keep shoes/bag in car
TV Room Set-Up	
• Couch with pillows	• Sit in a chair
• Reading newspaper	• Read while cycling
• Watching television	• Set alarm to stop watching
Support from Family Members	
• Time away from family	• Ask someone to walk with you
• Inactive children/spouse	• Be a role model
• Vacations in the car	• Camping and hiking

AT HOME. One of the first places to look for ways to be more active is where you live. Take a close look at your home to see how physical activity is encouraged or discouraged. Then, determine how to combat a sedentary lifestyle.

Doug owns a small mixed-breed dog named Pete. Pete stays in the apartment during the day while Doug is at work, so he's glad to see Doug when he comes home. Over the years, Doug has made it a habit to take Pete for a walk after dinner at about seven o'clock. Pete gets really excited when Doug takes out the leash. He knows it's time to go. If Doug gets busy and doesn't remember the walk, Pete reminds him by jumping and barking. Doug trained Pete to go for a walk; now Pete reminds Doug if he forgets. ●

9 Advantages of At-Home Exercise. Having exercise equip-ment in your home is no guarantee that you'll get fit or improve your health. You still have to do the work to get the benefit. However, it can be a tremen-dous boost to your physical activity program, for the following reasons.

- It's convenient. You don't have to drive to an-other location.
- It's comfortable. You don't have to change clothes. You could even exercise in your un-derwear.
- It's safe.
- Having the equipment in a visible location can remind you to be active.
- It's a one-time expense. Once you've invested in the equipment, there are usually no other ongoing costs.
- It may be able to be used by other family members.

- It's good for children to see the parents being active.
- It's possible to combine exercise with other activities, such as reading the newspaper or watching television.
- It's easy to include short bouts of exercise several times during the day.

A Primer on Buying Home Exercise Equipment. Many different types of exercise equipment are available for home use. Treadmills, stair-climbing machines, stationary cycles, rowing machines, and cross-country skiing machines are just a few of the types of cardiovascular fitness equipment you can buy.

Weight machines for strength training can also be purchased for home use. With such a wide variety of models and options offered within each type of equipment, how can you know you're making the best choice?

First, the exercise you want to do determines the type of equipment to shop for. So spend some time analyzing your needs and interests to decide on the type of equipment you want.

Next, and probably the most important step when buying exercise equipment, is to "try it before you buy it." You want to make certain that the equipment has the following features.

- Feels solid, not wobbly or tipsy.
- Can be adjusted to your specific body dimensions.
- Doesn't have parts that hit or pinch you or cramp your movements in an unnatural fashion.
- Operates smoothly and fluidly without excessive jerking or hitching.
- Isn't excessively noisy.
- Has adjustable resistance and/or speed so that you can vary your workouts.

When you're ready to try equipment, select a store that will let you test several different pieces of equipment at one visit. This will make it easier for you to comparison shop. When testing equipment, don't just try it for 30 seconds and make your decision. Do a complete workout on the equipment to get a feel for how it operates and how it feels when you are tired. As a rule, if a store won't let you try it, then take your business elsewhere. The ideal plan is to rent the brand and model of the equipment you want to buy and try it at home for a month or so.

Remember, you don't want your investment to end up functioning as a clothes rack or gathering dust in the garage because you made an impulse purchase. Use the checklist below to help you evaluate a variety of products.

EXERCISE EQUIPMENT CHECKLIST

	Product		
	A	B	C
Needs			
• Do you have any muscle or joint problems that should be taken into consideration?			
• Can you perform more than one type of exercise on the equipment? Do all varieties feel solid and smooth?			
• Do you have the skills to use the equipment?			
• How likely are you to get the results you want?			
• Is there any doubt about the safety of the equipment?			
• Can the piece be adjusted so that people of other sizes and fitness levels can use it?			

(continued)

	Product		
	A	B	C
Price, Warranty, and Service			
• How much does it cost?			
• Can you purchase the equipment used through the classified ads or a consignment store?			
• Is the equipment sturdy and likely to last for a number of years without a great deal of maintenance?			
• Does the equipment come with a warranty? What does it cover? For how long?			
• Is the manufacturer reputable? Does the manufacturer provide strong customer service?			
• If servicing is necessary, who do you call and what is it likely to cost you?			
• Are training materials or instructions provided, if needed?			
Requirements			
• Is electricity required to operate the equipment?			
• Will the equipment fit comfortably within the space available in your home?			
• Does it come assembled? Is it easy to assemble?			
• Is the equipment attractive?			
• Can you rent or lease it for a trial period to try it out for yourself before purchasing?			

Two of the most popular pieces of exercise equipment available for home purchase are stationary cycles and treadmills. Both simulate activities that are typically done outdoors but have the advantage of letting you stay active when the weather is bad.

When exercising indoors on a treadmill or stationary cycle, your body temperature will rise more rapidly than when you're exercising outdoors. This happens even if the temperature is the same. Why? Because outside there is air moving around your body to cool it. Expect to sweat more when exercising on equipment indoors. Place a fan nearby as a source of air and drink plenty of water if you sweat heavily.

POWER UP AT WORK. Most of us have very sedentary jobs. And work takes up a significant part of the day. What can you do to increase your physical activity during the workday? Here are a few ideas:

- Ask your company to sponsor fitness activities to encourage employees to be active.
- Brainstorm project ideas with a co-worker while taking a walk.
- Manage by walking around.
- Stand while talking on the phone.
- Walk while waiting for the plane at the airport.
- Make reservations at hotels with fitness centers or swimming pools when on business trips.
- Participate in a recreation league.
- Form a team to raise money for charity events.
- Walk down the hall to speak with someone rather than using the telephone.
- Schedule activity/stretch breaks when you plan meetings longer than one hour.
- Take along a jump rope in your suitcase when you travel. Jump and do calisthenics in your hotel room.
- Join a fitness center or Y near your work. Work out before or after work to avoid rush hour traffic, or drop by for a noon workout.

- Schedule your exercise time on your business calendar and treat it as any other important appointment.

Since every work situation is different, list other ways that you can be more active at work in the space below.

✓   **WAYS TO BE ACTIVE
         AT WORK**

- _____
- _____
- _____
- _____
- _____

AT PLAY. Play is important for good health. Adults need play and recreation. Look for opportunities to be active and have fun at the same time. Start with these ideas:

- Plan family outings and vacations that include physical activity (hiking, orienteering, backpacking, canoeing).
- See the sites in new cities by walking, jogging, or cycling. Take along enough money for a treat at a sidewalk cafe.
- Make a date with a friend to exercise.
- Wear fun clothing (bright colors, wild prints) when you exercise.
- Play your favorite music while exercising, something that motivates you.
- Dance—with someone or by yourself. Take dancing lessons.
- Join a recreational club that emphasizes activity.

List even more ways that you can build more activity into your recreational and leisure time. It's rare that anyone says they gave up exercise because it was too much fun!

✓	**WAYS TO BE ACTIVE** **AT PLAY**

- _____
- _____
- _____
- _____
- _____

---

21 Key Points to Choosing a Fitness Center

You certainly don't have to join a fitness center or go to a facility to exercise. For some people, though, it helps to have a special place to exercise. The staff, equipment, and educational resources there can help them reach their health and fitness goals.

Exercise and fitness are becoming so popular that an entire industry has emerged to service this need. In most cities there are several health clubs and fitness centers. The costs vary considerably. Some community recreation and fitness centers are available free and others cost as much as $100 per month.

If you're considering joining a health/fitness center, ask these questions to get the information you need to make an informed decision. Visit several clubs on a trial basis at the time of day you normally plan to exercise. Talk to current members to get their opinions about the facility and services.

- Is the location convenient to your home or work?
- Is the facility safe? Are surfaces for high-impact activities resilient?

- Are both the temperature and humidity level comfortable? Is there adequate ventilation?
- Are showers and lockers available? Is the facility clean and well maintained?
- What amenities (towels, shampoo, lotions, hair dryers, etc.) are provided?
- Is there ample space? Is the equipment or activity that interests you available at the time of day that you plan to visit the center?
- Is a childcare center available on site?
- Will an individualized exercise prescription be provided?
- Are a variety of fitness and health improvement programs offered?
- Is safety emphasized?
- Are programs in place to help you stay with your program?
- Do staff members hold appropriate certifications?
- Are staff healthy role models?
- Are fitness staff available to help you? Are they positive and supportive?
- Do you feel comfortable with the conditions of any waiver (such as a liability waiver) you are asked to sign before joining?
- Are warning signs and safety reminders posted in appropriate areas?
- Is a health screening performed as part of the orientation process?
- Are procedures in place to deal with emergencies?
- Is there a medical director for the center?
- What is the fee and what does it include?
- Is there a contract? What is the payment schedule?

If you're working out at a fitness center, you'll come in contact with professional exercise leaders. These people can make a significant contribution to your exercise program. They can:

- demonstrate new skills;
- monitor your movements for safety;
- help you make adjustments in your exercise program as you improve and progress;
- provide encouragement and recognition; and
- notice if you're absent and make you feel you were missed.

Ask the club manager about the specific qualifications and certifications of the fitness leaders in your club. The manager should be able to direct you to a leader that suits your needs.

How to Avoid Exercise Injuries

Before trying to increase your activity level and improve your cardiovascular fitness, you need to be aware of symptoms of overuse. Overuse symptoms are usually caused by trying to do too much too fast or by working too hard for too long. They're a common reason for dropping out of an exercise program in the early stages. Try to avoid these aches and pains by starting slowly and following the safety guidelines recommended in this book.

COMMON OVERUSE SYMPTOMS. Prevention is always the best practice. But if a problem occurs, take appropriate action so that you can get back on course as quickly as possible. Some of the most common overuse symptoms are discussed below.

Delayed Muscle Soreness. This soreness is not due to an injury. You usually feel this type of soreness within 24 to 72 hours after a strenuous activity. We don't know fully why this happens, but stretching, massage, and heat can make this type of soreness feel better.

Acute Muscle Soreness. Acute soreness can mean an injury. You may feel a burning sensation in the muscle due to a tear or rupture. These feelings usually appear suddenly when the muscle has been put under great or sudden strain. If the pain is severe or it continues for more than a few days, see your doctor. It's also a good idea to see a doctor for any injury that causes inflammation (redness to the skin) or severe swelling.

Blisters. Try to eliminate the cause of the blister. If you get a blister, pierce the edge of the blister with a sterilized needle. Be careful not to tear the skin after the blister has been drained. Treat the blister with an antiseptic ointment. Protect the area with an adhesive bandage and you can resume activity immediately.

Cramps. Cramps may be caused by an imbalance of sodium and potassium in the muscles. Stretching and massaging the muscle usually brings immediate relief. Taking appropriate time to warm up and cool down before and after activity can help prevent most cramps.

Knee Problems. Many knee problems are the result of previous injuries. Wearing proper shoes and exercising on soft, even surfaces helps avoid recurring knee problems. Also, to protect your knees, avoid activities such as tennis, basketball, or soccer that require sharp or quick turns.

Shin Splints. Shin splints are ˙sharp pains on the front part of the lower legs. There are many possible causes. Wearing shoes with plenty of cushion and support helps prevent shin splints. Unfortunately, rest is the only treatment for shin splints.

Low Back Pain. This is a very common complaint of adults today. It's usually caused by poor flexibility in the hamstrings and weak abdominal muscles. Poor posture also contributes to low back pain. Stretching and muscle building exercises can remedy this problem in most cases.

Tendonitis and Other Strains and Sprains. These problems have numerous causes. Some of them are: wearing improper or worn-out shoes; not warming up properly; and exercising on an uneven surface. Fortunately, the R.I.C.E. procedure described below works for most of these symptoms.

THE R.I.C.E. PROCEDURE. If you experience an overuse injury, follow the R.I.C.E procedure.

R = Rest. Stop the activity as soon as you notice any pain or discomfort. Continuing to exercise may just make it worse. "No pain, no gain" is just plain wrong. Rest for 24 hours or until there are no more symptoms of pain or injury.

I = Ice. Apply an ice pack immediately to a new injury. Ice decreases swelling and reduces pain. If there is swelling, apply ice off and on for 72 hours. Ice should never be placed directly on the skin, and the maximum time to apply each pack is 20 minutes. Using ice at bedtime isn't necessary unless the pain is severe.

C = Compression. Wrap the injury to reduce swelling. Start below the injury and wrap toward the heart. The wrap should be applied firmly, but not too tightly to cut off circulation. During the early stages when swelling is severe, loosen the wrap every half hour, then reapply.

E = Elevation. Elevate the injured part so that it is higher than the heart at all times initially (including during sleep). Continue to elevate as much as possible until swelling has subsided. Elevation uses gravity to prevent the pooling of blood and other fluids in the injured area.

See a doctor immediately if the:

- pain is severe;
- injured part can't be moved;
- pain continues for more than three days; or
- injury seems not to be healing after reasonable home treatment.

THE FOUR S'S OF EXERCISE SAFETY. You can minimize your risk of an overuse injury if you follow these four guidelines:

Stretch. Warm up for a few minutes by stretching the muscles and tendons that will be involved in the exercise you will do. If you're going to play tennis or golf, do shoulder and back stretches. If you're going to walk, jog, or cycle, stretch the thighs and calves. Examples of stretching exercises are provided on pages 162–163.

Shoes. You need the right kind of shoes for the activity that you'll be doing. See pages 179–180 for more information about selecting shoes.

Surface. High-impact activities, such as jumping rope, jogging, or running are particularly hard on your joints. So you want to make sure that the surface on which you are exercising has some "give" to it. In general, asphalt is better than concrete. Grass is better than asphalt (as long as the grass is even and free of holes or other hazards). The harder the surface, the more important it is to have shoes with adequate cushioning.

Also, most roads are built with a "crown." That's where the middle of the road is slightly higher than the sides. The crown allows water to run off into the gutters and storm drains. Be careful about jogging or running on streets with a high crown. The angled surface causes one leg to be higher than the other, which can lead to knee and hip problems over time.

Style. Learn to do any exercise or activity properly. Some people compromise their style or form to increase their intensity and speed. You could injure yourself or reduce the benefit you are getting for your effort. Get instructions or take lessons from an exercise professional to master new skills. Have someone recheck your style or technique from time to time.

Staying Active for a Lifetime

Most cars come with an extended warranty. If you take care of the car and get regular service checks, it will run well for a long time. Your heart and body can do the same—function well over your lifetime.

What causes some people to stay active while others seem to never get started or drop in and out of activity? People who can answer "yes" to the questions on the next page are most likely to stay active.

Tap into the Power of Supportive Relationships

Support is absolutely critical to adopting an activity program and staying with it. If you're married, try to get your spouse to join you in physical activity. You don't have to participate in the same type of activity or even exercise at the same time, but it's critical that you have the support of this important person. If your spouse is not supportive and tries to sabotage your efforts, it can be a serious barrier to staying active.

ARE YOU THE ACTIVE TYPE?

The Exerciser

YES   NO   Do you believe that your lifestyle habits affect your health?

YES   NO   Do you make physical activity a priority in your life and plan time for activity like any other important appointment?

YES   NO   Do you have other good health habits? (Are you a non-smoker? Do you always wear your seat belt and never drive after drinking alcohol?)

YES   NO   Do you generally feel in control of your life?

YES   NO   Are you self-motivated?

YES   NO   Are you monitoring your activity and tracking your progress?

YES   NO   Do you listen to your body to prevent overuse injuries?

YES   NO   Are you getting the results you want?

YES   NO   Do you spend your free time engaged in active rather than inactive pursuits?

The Environment

YES   NO   Is your work schedule generally stable and satisfactory?

YES   NO   Is it convenient for you to be active?

YES   NO   Can you integrate the activity into your daily routine?

YES   NO   Do you hae a special place to exercise that you like and where you feel safe?

YES   NO   Are there other people around you (family, friends, co-workers) who share your commitment to and interest in physical activity and health?

YES   NO   Do you have someone to exercise with (if that is your preference) or someone who is supportive of your physical activity?

The Exercise

YES   NO   Are you including aerobic, strength, and flexibility exercises for a balanced fitness program?

YES   NO   Do you enjoy your physical activities?

YES   NO   Is the intensity level appropriate for you (not too vigorous)?

YES   NO   Can you perform the exercise in more than one setting (not just a health club)?

YES   NO   Is your program safe?

YES   NO   Are you getting the results you want?

YES   NO   Is the activity one that you can perform over your lifetime?

Friends and co-workers can also be a great source of support for physical activity. Learn to ask for the type of support you need. Do you want someone to:

- Remind you to exercise?
- Ask about your progress?
- Participate with you regularly or occasionally?
- Allow you time to exercise by yourself (your special time alone)?
- Go with you to a special event (10K walk/run, bicycle race, swim meet)?
- Be understanding when you get up early to exercise in the morning?
- Spend time with the children while you exercise?
- Try not to ask you to change your exercise time?

List the types of support you need in the space on the next page.

Persons	What I Will Ask Them to Do
	•
	•
	•
	•

Barbara has learned that the key to staying with her swimming program is to go to the pool early in the morning. She leaves home at 5:30 every workday and heads for the club. Recently, Barbara started dating Bill. Early in the relationship she explained that she really enjoyed seeing him often. She also told him that it would help her if their dates on weeknights could end early enough so she could get up early in the morning for her swim. She was pleased to know that Bill was willing to support her exercise program. He even joins her at the club from time to time. They exercise together on weekends now and support each other's efforts to stay active. •

Your Child's Physical Activity Program

Help children develop good physical activity habits at an early age by setting a good example yourself. Limit the amount of television and substitute physical activity.

Stay involved in your child's physical education classes at school. Ask questions about:

- Frequency of classes and activity. Ideally, at least three days of vigorous activity will be offered.
- Class size. Physical education classes should be comparable in size to other classes.

- Curriculum. Instruction in lifetime fitness activities as well as team sports should be emphasized. Grades in physical education class should be based on knowledge and understanding of concepts as well as performance skills.
- Physical fitness assessments. Physical fitness should be measured on a regular basis to ensure that development is on track.
- Qualifications of the teacher. The teacher should hold appropriate certification in physical education and be an appropriate role model for students.

 Don took his son Mark along with him when he jogged almost from the time Mark was born. He'd put the baby in the stroller and off they'd go. As Mark grew, he continually saw his dad engaged in various fitness activities. When Mark could ride a bicycle, he'd ride along as Don jogged or biked.

Mark grew up and is now married. Physical activity is a priority for him. In fact, Don and Mark frequently run 10K's together on weekends. Mark's going to be a father soon. Don is planning to purchase one of the baby strollers designed for joggers as a gift for Mark and the baby. ●

Exercise Facts and Fallacies

I've always been a couch potato. It's too late for me to change.

It's never too late to change. Studies show that sedentary people who adopt an active lifestyle receive a significant health benefit even if they've been sedentary for most of their lives. Changing from being inactive to being active is as important as changing other important risk factors for cardio-vascular disease. These risk factors include quitting smoking, lowering blood pressure and blood cholesterol levels to within healthy ranges, and losing weight if overweight.

The best thing about changing your activity habits is that you're adding something positive to your life instead of taking something away.

I'm too old to be active.

Nonsense! Physical activity is a key factor in healthy aging. The physiological decline associated with aging may actually be the result of inactivity. More than 40 percent of people over the age of 65 report no leisure time physical activity. Less than a third participate in regular moderate physical activity, such as walking or gardening, and less than 10 percent engage routinely in vigorous physical activity.

Some studies have shown that increased levels of physical activity are associated with a reduced incidence of coronary heart disease, hypertension, non-insulin-dependent diabetes, colon cancer, and depression and anxiety. All of these diseases are common in older adults. Increased physical activity increases bone mineral content, which reduces the risk of fractures. Activity increases muscle strength and may also improve balance and coordination. These factors may reduce the likelihood of falls in older people. Perhaps the most important benefit of physical activity is that it enables people to retain their independence throughout the later years of life. One study suggests that people with higher levels of physical fitness and physical activity are less likely to develop the functional limitations often associated with aging. These include problems with personal care such as bathing, dressing, and feeding.

Women don't benefit as much as men from physical activity.

Women respond to exercise and activity in generally the same physiological and biochemical way as men. They also derive the same health benefits. Yet, with respect to world records in major athletic events, performances by men are in all respects better than by women.

What explains this difference? Women are generally shorter and lighter than men. They have more fatty tissue and less muscle. The absolute strength of females is only about two-thirds that of men. Women have fewer total red blood cells and about 15 percent less hemoglobin.

Women get big muscles when they exercise.

The male hormone, testosterone, is responsible for muscle bulkiness in males. This hormone is present in women, but in quantities one-tenth that of men. Women who have participated in an intense weight training program for several months have shown significant increases in strength. However, their increase in muscle size might be relatively small.

Women benefit significantly from weight bearing exercise, especially after menopause. As women and men grow older, there is a tendency for bones to lose calcium. Individuals who experience severe bone loss are said to have osteoporosis. Bones, like muscles, get stronger and thicker the more they are exercised. Many exercises slow down the bone loss process. These include weight training, walking, and running.

Genetic factors influence your health and fitness, not how much you exercise.

It's true that the traits you inherit from your family are known to influence both your health and physical fitness performance. You must accept that there are some characteristics about your body that you cannot change even though you are dedicated to your exercise program. Also, some diseases, such as cardiovascular disease and breast cancer, seem to be linked to family history. While you should be aware of these genetic influences, you shouldn't be discouraged from exercising. Physical activity can still help improve and maintain your body and your fitness level. You may not have what it takes to be an elite athlete, but you can improve your health and enjoy the fun of activities.

Jogging is the best exercise.

No single exercise is best. Jogging can be an excellent choice for some people, but it's not for everyone. The key to staying active is to select an exercise or activity that you like to do and that you want to do.

HIGHLIGHTS ────────────────────────────

Exercise and Your Heart

Regular physical activity is as important to keeping your heart healthy as brushing and flossing is to keeping your teeth healthy. You don't have to brush and floss all day—just after meals. You don't have to run a marathon—just work some moderate physical activity into your day, every day. It's one of the most important keys to a healthy heart.

CHAPTER SIX

Clearing the Air— How to Quit Smoking and Start Living

 ### The Fundamentals of Air Quality

Have you ever passed a car on the highway with black smoke coming out of its tailpipe? If you listened closely, the engine was probably sputtering and choking. A car like that is likely to need major repairs, and the owner will be out a lot of money if the condition is neglected for too long. Too bad, because most major repairs of that type can be avoided.

In the same way, your heart and lungs can't operate very efficiently if you smoke. Smokers have a greater risk for developing heart disease, stroke, cancer, emphysema, and chronic bronchitis. Smoking slows you down and costs you a lot of money, much more than just the cost of the cigarettes. In fact, over a lifetime, smokers have significantly higher medical bills than non-smokers. In this chapter, you'll find out how to quit smoking for good—and how to keep others' smoke out of your life.

211

Are You Ready to Quit?

Most smokers know they should quit, and they want to. Some have quit before, maybe several times, then started smoking again. Being ready to quit is critically important in quitting for good. If you're currently a smoker, or have a friend or family member who's a smoker, this quiz will help determine if this is a good time to quit.

 STOP SMOKING READINESS QUIZ

Are you ready to quit? Let's find out. Circle "Yes" if you agree with the statement; "No" if you disagree.

YES	NO	I know that smoking is harmful to my health.
YES	NO	Quitting will be difficult, but I really want to try.
YES	NO	I can get support from my family and friends.
YES	NO	I have tried to quit before.
YES	NO	Quitting is something I want to do for myself.
YES	NO	I can make quitting smoking my top priority for the next three to 12 months.
YES	NO	I am confident that I will be able to stay off cigarettes.

If you answered "Yes" to four or more of these statements, you are probably ready to quit. If you answered "No" to four or more statements, this may not be a good time for you to quit smoking. That's okay for right now. You'll be much more likely to succeed in quitting for good if you do it when *you're* ready.

But don't forget about quitting. Review this quiz and the following "Ten Big Benefits of Quitting Smoking" every few months. At some point in the future, you may be ready to quit. Even if you're not ready now, you could benefit from reading the remainder of this section to learn more about the smoking habit and options for quitting.

 ## Ten Big Benefits of Quitting Smoking

Quitting smoking carries major and immediate health benefits for men and women of all ages, even those in the older age groups. The benefits apply both to healthy people and to those already suffering from smoking-related diseases.

Experts agree that stopping smoking is the single most important step that smokers can take to increase the quantity and quality of their lives. The message is simple: Add years to your life, and life to your years. Here is a list of some of the health benefits of quitting smoking.

- Within 12 hours of quitting, your body begins to heal itself. The levels of carbon monoxide and nicotine in your system decline rapidly, and your heart and lungs will begin to repair the damage caused by cigarette smoke.
- Within a few days, your senses of smell and taste will improve. The cough associated with smoking will disappear, and your digestive system will return to normal. It will be easier to climb a hill or a flight of stairs without becoming winded or dizzy.
- Soon you will be feeling better about yourself and in control of your life. You'll enjoy being free of the mess, smell, inconvenience, and expense of smoking.
- After quitting smoking, regardless of how long or how much you've smoked, your risk of heart disease rapidly declines. Three years after quit-

ting, the risk of death from heart disease and stroke for people who smoked a pack a day or less is almost the same as for people who have never smoked. The risk of death from cancer, chronic bronchitis, and emphysema is also significantly reduced.

- It's never too late. Men and women who quit at ages 65 to 69 increase their life expectancy by one year.
- Even for people who are sick, quitting can help. For people with heart disease, quitting reduces the risk of repeat heart attacks and death from heart disease by 50 percent or more. For people with ulcers, quitting smoking reduces the risk of recurrence and improves short-term healing.
- If all women quit smoking during pregnancy, about five percent of deaths among newborn infants could be prevented.
- Women who stop smoking before becoming pregnant or during the first trimester of pregnancy reduce their risk of having a low birthweight baby to that of women who have never smoked.
- It takes female smokers longer to get pregnant than nonsmokers. Women who quit smoking before trying to get pregnant are as likely to get pregnant as women who have never smoked.
- People who quit smoking are more likely to exercise regularly than smokers. Exercise may help new quitters deal with withdrawal symptoms and stay off cigarettes. It's also critical to weight management efforts.

Methods for Quitting Smoking

If you're ready to quit or know someone who is, it's important to think about the method of quitting most likely to work. Years of research and experience show that there is no one sure way to quit, but some of the more common methods are discussed below.

GOING IT ALONE—THE SELF-HELP APPROACH. Many smokers quit on their own or with very little outside help. They may read educational booklets, watch videos, or use quit kits. A variety of self-help programs are available through voluntary health organizations, such as the American Heart Association, the American Cancer Society, the American Lung Association, and other groups. Your doctor may be able to recommend self-help materials to help you quit smoking on your own.

Self-help programs are attractive to many smokers because:

- they offer privacy and convenience;
- the program can be completed at a flexible pace on your own schedule;
- you don't have to attend meetings; and
- they are free or cost very little.

There are four steps that are common to many self-help programs for quitting. These self-help suggestions can be combined into a variety of programs.

First Step. List the positive reasons why you want to quit smoking. Post these reasons where you'll be sure to see them. Read the list daily. Periodically, write down new reasons why you're glad you quit.

My Reasons for Quitting:

-
-
-
-
-

I'm Glad I Quit Because:

- _____
- _____
- _____
- _____
- _____

Wrap your cigarette pack with a copy of the "Smoking Habits Log" from Appendix A and secure with a rubber band. Each time you smoke, write down the time of day, what you're doing, and how you feel using a scale from 1 to 5. Then rewrap the pack. This exercise will help you understand why you smoke.

Second Step. Keep reading your list of reasons for quitting, and add to it if possible. Don't carry matches, and keep your cigarettes some distance away. Each day, try to smoke fewer cigarettes, eliminating those least or most important cigarettes (whichever works best).

Third Step. Continue with the second step's instructions. Don't buy a new pack until you finish the one you're smoking, and never buy a carton. Change brands twice during the week, each time choosing a brand lower in tar and nicotine. Try to stop smoking for 48 hours sometime during this step.

Fourth Step. Quit smoking entirely. Increase your physical activity. Avoid situations you most closely associate with smoking. Find a substitute for cigarettes. Do deep breathing exercises whenever you get the urge to smoke.

USING NICOTINE CHEWING GUM OR PATCH. Addiction to nicotine makes it very difficult for some smokers to give up cigarettes. Nicotine gum and the nicotine patch contain enough nicotine to reduce the urge for cigarettes. These items are prescription drugs, so you must see your doctor to get them.

If you decide to use the nicotine gum, you'll start off chewing one piece every time you feel the need to smoke. Over time, you chew fewer pieces of gum, and you gradually become less dependent on nicotine. If you use the nicotine patch, you will apply the patch to your skin. A small amount of nicotine will be released slowly and absorbed through your skin.

The major advantage of using these products is that they work directly on the physiological addiction to nicotine. There are disadvantages, however. The cost may be a problem for you. You must not continue to smoke if you are using either of these products, and there is a limit to how long you can use these methods. It is strongly recommended that nicotine gum and the nicotine patch be used in combination with other programs that help break your psychological dependence on cigarettes.

Answer the questions below to discover your level of smoking addiction. If you answer "yes" to more than two questions, a nicotine substitute may help you gradually break your addiction.

HOW ADDICTED ARE YOU?

___ Do you smoke your first cigarette within 30 minutes of waking up in the morning?

___ Do you smoke one pack (20 cigarettes) or more each day?

___ At times when you can't smoke or when you don't have a cigarette, do you crave one?

___ Is it hard for you to go more than a few hours without smoking?

___ When you are sick enough to stay in bed, do you still smoke?

GETTING HELP FROM A GROUP PROGRAM. Some people benefit from the support of a group program to help them quit. Members of the group can provide counseling and a supportive environment for one another. Some of these programs are quite successful, but the cost and the time required to attend meetings may prevent some smokers from joining groups. Many companies that offer "smoke-free" environments will provide smoking cessation programs for their employees who smoke. The convenience of participating during or after work, the opportunity for support from co-workers, and the possible reduced cost or financial incentive to quit are all advantages of stop-smoking programs at work. Inquire about these types of programs at your worksite.

A WALK ON THE WILD SIDE—USING CONDITIONING METHODS. The two most common conditioning methods used to help smokers quit are: rapid smoking (inhaling every few seconds) and satiation (smoking two or three times as many cigarettes as normal). These quitting methods condition smokers to feel sick when they think about smoking.

Unfortunately, these methods usually show limited results, and they are among the most expensive available. In addition, there are possible health risks associated with these methods. Be sure to talk to your doctor before using any conditioning method.

TRYING IT 24 HOURS A DAY—THE LIVE-IN APPROACH. If you are a heavy smoker and strongly addicted to nicotine, you may benefit from a live-in stop-smoking program. These programs are usually operated by health professionals in hospitals or clinics and seem to be quite effective.

In these programs, you live in a non-smoking environment for several days or weeks. While there, you participate in quit-smoking activities that may include education, group support, counseling, fitness, exercise, and weight management. These programs are very expensive. Also, some participants find it extremely difficult to return to their normal environment when the program is completed.

USING THE POWER OF SUGGESTION: HYPNOSIS. Only licensed psychiatrists, psychologists, or accredited social workers are qualified to perform hypnosis therapy. In this method, the therapist hypnotizes you and gives you suggestions to help you stop smoking. The suggestions are designed to help you relax when you feel the urge to smoke, feel good about the times you didn't smoke, and feel badly about the times you slipped and smoked.

If hypnosis works for you, these suggestions will stay in your mind even after the session ends and will help you avoid smoking in the future. Because it usually takes several sessions to improve your chances of quitting, this method is time-consuming and expensive.

TRYING ACUPUNCTURE. Certain nerve endings near the surface of the skin are thought to be associated with the urge to smoke. Acupuncture treatment for smoking consists of inserting needles or staples into the skin near these surface nerves. It is relatively painless.

You usually need multiple treatments to increase the chances of quitting smoking, and treatments can be expensive. Also, acupuncture may have only a psychological effect and not a true physical effect.

USING OVER-THE-COUNTER STOP-SMOKING PRODUCTS. There are numerous over-the-counter products that claim to be the easy way to stop smoking. A few examples include special filters for cigarettes, pills,

non-nicotine gum, throat lozenges, smokeless cigarettes, mouth sprays, electronic devices, and too many
others to name individually. Very few of these methods have been shown to be effective in helping smokers quit.

 ## Questions to Ask About Any Stop-Smoking Program

If you're considering a program to help you stop
smoking, be sure to ask questions about the program
before you make a final decision, especially if there
are costs involved.

- How convenient is the program for you?
- What educational or behavioral modification
  components are included? Look for the following
  features in the program:
    a plan or contract for quitting that includes a
        quit date;
    skills for coping with the urge to smoke and
        withdrawal symptoms;
    ways to involve others and build support;
    ways to identify triggers to smoke and plan for
        high-risk situations;
    ways to avoid gaining weight;
    strategies for dealing with slips; and
    rewards for not smoking.
- In determining success rate, what definition of
  quitting is used? (You'll want a strict definition,
  such as staying off cigarettes completely.)
- How many participants are enrolled in the
  program?
- What are the quit rates for program participants
  at 6 to 12 months after the end of the program?

How to Get Support for Quitting

It's not easy to quit smoking, especially if smoking has been a habit for a long time. Heavy smokers often need a lot of support to help them quit. If you're a smoker, ask someone to help you quit or to quit with you. Tell them specifically how they can help. You may want them to:

- talk about the reasons for quitting;
- analyze previous attempts to quit and what led to a return to smoking;
- help plan strategies to deal with triggers to smoke and withdrawal symptoms;
- give encouragement and praise; and
- just be there to talk or visit.

If you are trying to help someone quit smoking, keep these points in mind.

- Don't be disappointed if the smoker only quits for a few days. Give praise for having the courage to try. Emphasize that it's important to learn from the experience in order to be better prepared for the next try.
- Let your smoker know you care, but be prepared for a cold shoulder at times. Some smokers want to be left alone.
- Know the possible symptoms associated with withdrawal from smoking: anxiety, headaches, anger, poor concentration. Be patient and remind the smoker that the symptoms don't last. Encourage the smoker to think of these symptoms as signs of recovery.
- Don't suggest an activity that would put the smoker in a high-risk situation. For example, don't suggest going to a club to hear music if

that's a place where he or she did a lot of smoking.
- Be there!

About Gaining Weight

It's true. Gaining weight is a common fear and problem for people who stop smoking. The average weight gain after quitting is just five pounds, and only 3.5 percent of those who quit gain more than 20 pounds after quitting.

The health benefits of quitting far exceed any risk from the average 5-pound weight gain that may follow quitting. *It would take a 75-pound weight gain to offset the health benefits that a normal smoker gains by quitting.*

Of course, you don't have to automatically gain weight when you quit. You can make weight management a part of your plan to stop smoking (see "How to Get Rid of Your Spare Tire," pages 230–257).

WEIGHT MANAGEMENT TIPS

- Plan menus carefully, counting calories and fat grams.
- Have low-calorie foods on hand for nibbling.
- Increase your physical activity to burn more calories.
- A walking program helps with weight management and takes your mind off the desire to smoke.
- Weigh yourself no more frequently than once a week to monitor your progress.

How to Stay a Non-Smoker

You can use many different strategies and skills to help you fight the urge to smoke. Among the most important is reviewing your list of reasons for wanting to quit smoking. Sometimes all you need to do is gently remind yourself of the good things you will get as a result of not smoking.

Another skill is to anticipate high-risk situations, such as pressure from the boss, frustration, or becoming too tired. Recognizing these problems early can help you develop specific strategies to cope with them when they're triggered.

Warren, a 28-year-old bachelor, was on his way home from a weekend at the beach. He was pleased with how well it had gone. Warren had just stopped smoking after nine years of the habit, and he hadn't been as irritable or jumpy as he had feared.

As the traffic got heavy, he became frustrated. He was alone in the car—no one to talk to—and caught in a traffic jam. He reached in his pocket where he used to keep his cigarettes. Of course, none were there. Then he spotted a gas station at the corner. "Maybe I'll pull off the road and buy a pack of cigarettes," he thought. After a minute of inner struggle, he pulled off the road and took a stretch break instead. This gave him a chance to review once again all of the reasons why he had quit smoking. ●

Four Reasons to Avoid Secondhand Tobacco Smoke

You don't have to be a smoker to be affected by smoke. Environmental tobacco smoke (secondhand or passive smoke) is estimated to cause the deaths of over 40,000 non-smokers each year. Most of these deaths are caused by heart disease. Other reasons to avoid secondhand smoke are:

- tobacco smoke can aggravate asthmatic conditions and impaired blood circulation;

- children exposed to secondhand smoke have more colds, pneumonia, bronchitis, and other respiratory problems;
- pregnant women who smoke have a higher rate of miscarriage, stillbirths, premature births, and complications of pregnancy than nonsmokers; and
- pregnant nonsmokers who are exposed to cigarette smoke deliver low birth weight babies more often than those who were not exposed to cigarette smoke.

Use the following quiz to help assess your risk for secondhand smoke at home and at work. Answer the questions below, choosing only one response for each statement.

To score your quiz:

- Give yourself 0 points for each "a" answer.
- Give yourself 1 point for each "b" answer.
- Give yourself 2 points for each "c" answer.
- Give yourself 4 points for each "d" answer.

Add your points for
- Work— _____ points
  +
- Home— _____ points
  _____ Total Score

On which items did you select "c" or "d"? ____

If your total score was:

0–8　　You are probably not breathing in much secondhand smoke. Look to see if you selected "c" or "d" for any statements. Think of ways to reduce your exposure to smoke in these places.

CLEARING THE AIR QUIZ

At Work	At Home
1. I can smell cigarette smoke when I'm at my work station. a. Never b. sometimes c. Frequently d. Always	5. I allow friends and family to smoke in my house. a. Never b. Sometimes c. Frequently d. Always
2. The smoking policy at work is: a. Smoke-free (no smoking in the building or on other company property, such as cars) b. Smoking only in specially ventilated smoking rooms c. Smoking restricted to break rooms, cafeteria, or other areas shared by smokers and nonsmokers d. Unrestricted smoking	6. Number of people in my household who smoke. a. None b. Just me c. Me and one other person d. Me and two or more other people
3. I take breaks with co-workers who smoke. a. Never b. Sometimes c. Frequently d. Always	7. I allow friends or family to smoke while I am in the car. a. Never b. Sometimes c. Frequently d. Always
4. I attend meetings where people are allowed to smoke. a. Never b. Sometimes c. Frequently d. Always	8. I sit in the smoking section when eating out at restaurants or when traveling on long plane trips. a. Never b. Sometimes c. Frequently d. Always

9–16   You could be inhaling a large amount of secondhand smoke. If you're a smoker, this amount is added to what you take in directly when you smoke. Review your scores again. Is your score higher for work or for home? This will give you a good idea where to start to reduce your exposure to secondhand smoke.

17–32   You are being exposed to large amounts of secondhand cigarette smoke. Is work or home the main culprit? Or both? Identify one statement for which you selected "c" or "d." Plan ways to reduce your exposure to cigarette smoke in this place. When you have mastered this change, pick another area to change.

I will reduce my exposure to secondhand smoke at _____ by doing the following:

* _____
* _____
* _____

 Your Children—Are They at Risk?

Your children learn about smoking from a variety of sources. Are they getting mixed messages? Are they at risk of becoming smokers, or are they in danger of becoming ill from secondhand smoke?

WHEN PARENTS SMOKE AT HOME. Studies have shown that children of smoking parents, especially infants, have more lung illnesses (bronchitis and pneumonia) than children of parents who do not smoke. Parents who smoke have a greater tendency to cough, which is more likely to spread germs and expose children to chest illnesses. Also, children are forced to breathe their parents' cigarette smoke in the closed environment of the home. Even if the parents are nonsmokers, children can be exposed to smoke if the parents' friends who visit are allowed to smoke around the children.

Even though adults are quitting smoking in large numbers, children are continuing to start. Children whose parents smoke are likely to become smokers. More than three million of the 54 million smokers in the United States are teenagers. The most shocking fact is that more girls than boys are smoking cigarettes.

Are your children exposed to secondhand smoke? Use this quiz to find out. Answer the questions below, choosing only one response for each statement.

CHILDREN AT RISK QUIZ

1. I . . .
    a. have never smoked or have quit smoking.
    b. smoke, but not in the presence of my children.
    c. smoke in the presence of my children.
    d. buy cigarettes for my children who smoke.
2. Smoking materials (cigarettes, lighters, ashtrays) are left out where my children can handle them.
    a. Never
    b. Sometimes
    c. Frequently
    d. Always
3. I allow friends or relatives to smoke around my children.
    a. Never
    b. Sometimes
    c. Frequently
    d. Always
4. I allow my teenager(s) to smoke in the house.
    a. Never (or no teenager at home)
    b. Sometimes
    c. Frequently
    d. Always

5. My children and I are uncomfortable discussing the hazards of smoking.
   a. Never
   b. Sometimes
   c. Frequently
   d. Always
6. I feel unprepared to answer my children's questions about smoking.
   a. Never
   b. Sometimes
   c. Frequently
   d. Always

If your total score was:

0–6   Congratulations! You are providing a home environment that helps support a smoke-free lifestyle. Still, work on any problem areas by identifying statements to which you answered "c" or "d." Also, be prepared to talk openly with your child if he or she shows an interest in trying to smoke.

7–14   Your children may be exposed to influences at home that could make it more likely that they would pick up the smoking habit. The statements for which you selected "c" or "d" are problem areas. Focus on changing one or two problem areas at first.

15–24   Your home environment does not appear to support a smoke-free lifestyle. This may confuse your children since they are probably learning in school to avoid smoking. Review your answers. See how you could provide a home environment that helps your children to choose a smoke-free life.

I will reduce my children's exposure to smoke by doing the following:

* _____
* _____
* _____

AT SCHOOL AND IN THE COMMUNITY. Do your part to support school and community efforts to discourage young people from smoking. Parents should tell school officials they expect enforcement of "no smoking" rules and that they are not in favor of special areas being set aside as student smoking areas. Support laws to prohibit stores from selling tobacco products to minors.

Most schools now are required to teach children about the dangers of smoking and how to resist peer pressure to smoke. But schools can't solve the problem alone. Parents and teachers must work together. Providing a good role model for children is important.

HIGHLIGHTS ————————————————————

Calling It Quits

Since the 1960's, millions of Americans have quit smoking. Millions more have demanded a smoke-free atmosphere in workplaces, airplanes, grocery stores, restaurants, and public buildings. They know that it's time to call it quits—for good.

CHAPTER SEVEN

How to Get Rid of Your Spare Tire

 The Fine Art of Losing Weight

As you drive around in your car, having a spare tire in the trunk is a necessity. Most of the time you don't need it. But when you have a flat it sure is nice to know that you're prepared. In fact, it could be considered hazardous not to have a spare tire.

But having a "spare tire" around your waist *is* hazardous. Research has shown that extra body fat, especially body fat stored in the waist area, increases risk for high blood pressure, high blood cholesterol, and diabetes. As you know, these factors increase your overall risk of having a heart attack or stroke. Excess body fat may also increase your risk for certain types of cancer and problems such as arthritis.

Having excess body fat will increase your overall body weight. The following pages describe how your body fat is formed and why maintaining a healthful body fat (and body weight) level is important. Also included are recommended weight levels and skills for getting rid of the spare tire if you need to.

Body Fat—A Delicate Balancing Act

In today's weight-conscious society, fat has become a "four-letter" word. While too much fat can increase risk for a lot of health problems, it's also hard on your social life. The prevailing attitude is, "thin is in." But you need *a little* body fat because it performs several essential functions. It:

- cushions internal organs,
- helps maintain hormone levels,
- helps store fat-soluble vitamins, and
- stores extra energy for times when you do not eat enough food.

When the gas gauge in your car points to "E," you know that you're going to stop dead on the highway unless you get to a gas station quickly. Your body, on the other hand, carries body fat, an energy reserve. So when you're hungry and can't get food right away, you don't just "stop dead on the highway." You burn your own body fat until you can get something to eat.

Your body works on a finely tuned energy balance system. Every second of every day, it uses energy to perform basic life-sustaining functions (pumping the heart, moving the lungs, fueling chemical reactions within cells). This is called your basal metabolism. Many factors, listed below, affect how much energy is burned (calories) in maintaining basic body metabolism.

- *Body size.* The larger the body, the higher the basal metabolic rate. This is because a larger body has more lean tissue than a smaller body. Lean tissue includes muscle, bones, and organs.
- *Genetics.* Research has shown that people within the same family tend to have similar metabolic rates.

- *Sex*. Males usually have higher metabolic rates, due mostly to more lean tissue.
- *Age*. Here again, lean tissue plays a role in determining basal metabolism. After reaching adulthood, the amount of lean tissue gradually decreases, thereby decreasing basal metabolism. You can slow this rate of decline by slowing the rate of lean tissue loss through physical activity.
- *Weight status*. Losing weight often decreases your metabolic rate. That's because some of any weight loss will be lean tissue. Also, restricting your calories may cause your metabolic rate to slow down in an attempt to "conserve" what little energy it is receiving.

Each of these factors plays a role in how many calories the body burns while you're at rest. Even if all these factors were identical in two different people, there would still probably be a slight difference. Scientists aren't sure yet what accounts for these differences.

Another way your body burns calories is a process called thermogenesis. Literally, this means "the creation of heat." But unlike basal metabolism, thermogenesis only occurs when specific conditions exist. They are:

- *Exposure to cold temperatures*. The body generates more heat to keep itself warm in cold environments.
- *Food intake*. The body produces heat when it goes through the many chemical reactions that digest, absorb, and store food. This uses only a small amount of your total daily energy.

You cannot easily change your body's basal metabolism or thermogenesis. You can, however, control the amount of energy your body uses to move around every day. The more active you are, the more calories you burn. It's as simple as that.

Our energy comes from only one place: the foods and beverages we consume. And this is where the balancing act comes into play.

- If you take in more energy (calories) than your body needs to move around, the extra energy is stored as fat. This causes weight gain.
- If your energy expenditure is greater than the energy intake from food and beverages, then your body will have to call on its energy reserves (body fat) to make up the difference. As body fat stores are diminished, your body weight goes down.
- If your calorie intake is equal to your energy expenditure, then body fat is neither added nor lost. Your weight will remain stable.

Why Are We So Fat?

Recent studies show that in spite of all the attention paid to staying slim and trim, American adults are actually becoming heavier. As many as 36 percent of women and 34 percent of men are overweight. To understand it, you must look into our collective history.

Many thousands of years ago, as the first humans were learning to survive, they were at the mercy of nature. Droughts and poor hunting conditions often brought famine and disease. Given these conditions, the human body became adept at storing food energy (as body fat) during the abundant times so that it could survive during the lean times.

As humans learned to harness nature by domesticating animals and tilling the soil, the most developed nations created an abundant food supply and experienced few, if any, periods of famine. And, now, with the "miracles" of modern technology (cars, washing machines, lawn mowers, computers, etc.) we have drastically reduced our daily energy expenditure. All this has happened in a relatively short period of time, so the human body has had little time to adapt to lots of food and little physical work. The result is a population that is more prone to having excess body fat and, consequently, being overweight.

Measuring Body Fat—Easier Said than Done

So what is a healthy body fat level? Unfortunately, scientists don't really know. What we do know is that people with higher body fat levels are at higher risk for developing health problems. At the same time, just because you have a high body fat level doesn't mean you will develop these problems. In fact, there are people with a high body fat level who are perfectly healthy. And there are people with a low body fat level who have high blood cholesterol, high blood pressure, and a host of other health problems.

One of the reasons an "ideal" body fat level has not been determined is that body fat is fairly difficult to measure. It is especially difficult to collect body fat data on a large number of people.

scientific methods. Measuring body fat accurately requires precise equipment, special training, and standardized protocols. Several of the methods currently available include the following.

- *Underwater weighing.* A person is weighed on land and again underwater in a special tank. Body fat is more buoyant than lean tissue. Thus, the more fat a person has, the greater the difference between the two weights. Special mathematical equations are used to estimate the amount of body fat. Because of the cumbersome equipment, this method is mostly used in research centers.

- *Skinfold measurements*. Since much of our body fat is right below the surface of our skin, "the pinch an inch" guideline can be put into practice. Special calipers are used to measure the thickness of skinfolds at several different sites on the body. Again, measurements are used in special equations to estimate body fat level. These measurements are much easier to do than underwater weighing, so they are used more frequently by dietitians, athletic coaches, and health club workers. Like any tool, however, this method is only as good as the training of the person using it.

- *Bioelectrical impedance*. A relatively new tool, this method attaches small electrodes on a person's wrist and one ankle. A small (you don't even feel it) charge is sent from one electrode to the other. The special equipment measures the current and can estimate the amount of body fat from that. This method does not seem to be very accurate for the very thin or the very fat and is somewhat dependent on the body's hydration state.

- *Circumferences*. Body fat can be estimated by taking measurements at certain parts of your body (waist, upper arm, chest, thigh, hips). Still, the equations that use circumferences to estimate body fat level are not as accurate as some of the other measurements. One of the best ways to use circumference measurements is to measure your waist circumference and your hip circumference and then calculate the ratio between the two (divide your waist measurement by your hip measurement). For example, if a man had a 44-inch waist and a 36-inch hip measurement, he'd have a waist-to-hip ratio of 1.2. By contrast, a man with a 33-inch waist and a 36-inch hip measurement would have a waist-to-hip ratio of about .9. The smaller the ratio, the less fat the man carries. While this does not tell you *how much* body fat you have, it does show where most of it is located. As discussed earlier on pages 10–11, body shape is also a contributing factor to heart disease risk.

It's important to realize that none of these methods directly measures body fat—they simply generate calculated estimates. Also, as mentioned earlier, there are no standardized recommendations for a healthy body fat for any of these methods. So the best way to use these tools is to assess change over time. This can be done by having a person skilled in a particular method periodically take measurements. Several measurements by the same technician using the same method over time can detect whether body fat is increasing, decreasing, or staying about the same.

The method most people use is measuring body weight. The trouble is, you cannot estimate the amount of body fat you have simply by knowing your body weight. For example, it's possible for two people to be the same height and weight, yet have very different amounts of body fat. Or the same person could weigh the same throughout his or her lifetime, but be gradually increasing in body fat.

Joey was a veteran of the Korean War. As a young lieutenant, he cut a splendid picture in his uniform—fit, trim, and eager.

Joey's unit was planning a reunion, and he was looking forward to showing everybody how little he had changed over the years. Joey knew for certain that, unlike most of the other guys, he was still at his

enlistment weight. But when he tried on his old uniform, he was surprised and dismayed to discover the
buttons and buttonholes gapped by several inches!

Joey learned later that even though he had not
gained weight since his Army days, he had gradually
lost lean tissue (mostly muscle mass) and gained
enough fat mass to keep his weight stable. While his
weight remained the same, his body fat level increased
over time. ●

Despite these problems, measuring weight is the
quickest and easiest method for getting a general idea
of how fat you are. If your body weight is high, you
are probably carrying around extra weight as body fat.

So, how high is too high? Scientists simply don't
know. But they are trying to develop more precise
ways to describe a healthy weight. In the meantime,
use the guidelines on the next page to help judge if
your weight is healthy.

This height and weight table probably looks a little
different from others you've seen. Instead of having
separate tables for men and women, it incorporates
both by having a broad weight range for each height.
The higher weight at each height typically applies to
men. Men usually have larger frames and more muscle
mass. Women should strive to stay on the lower end
of each weight range.

Having two different age categories is based on
research that shows weighing a little more is not
unhealthy in older men and women. Still, if you are
able to comfortably maintain your weight at the lower
weight range, don't use the weight ranges for older
adults as an excuse to put on a few extra pounds.

There are several other methods for assessing body
fat and body weight. One is to come face-to-face with
the "naked truth." That is, simply stand naked in
front of a full length mirror. Is the "spare tire" pretty

evident? Do you look different from the way you would like to look? Be careful not to be too critical. Not everyone was born to be a fashion model!

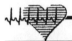

Height (Without Shoes)	Weight in Pounds (Without Clothes)	
	19–34 years	35 years +
5'0"	97–128	108–135
5'1"	101–132	111–143
5'2"	104–137	115–148
5'3"	107–141	119–152
5'4"	111–146	122–157
5'5"	114–150	126–162
5'6"	118–155	130–167
5'7"	121–160	134–172
5'8"	125–164	138–178
5'9"	129–169	142–183
5'10"	132–174	146–188
5'11"	136–179	151–194
6'0"	140–184	155–199
6'1"	144–189	159–205
6'2"	148–195	164–210
6'3"	152–200	168–216
6'4"	156–205	173–222
6'5"	160–211	177–228
6'6"	164–216	182–234

YOUR OPTIMAL WEIGHT

GUESSING YOUR BEST WEIGHT. You probably have a past weight in mind, a weight at which you felt your best. At that weight, you had lots of get-up-and-go all day long, didn't obsess about food, and didn't have to be a workout fanatic to maintain it.

It all comes down to what is a good weight for you. The best weight for you is one at which you look good, feel good, and have low health risks (such as high blood pressure and high blood cholesterol). It also is a weight that you can easily maintain over the years.

Managing Your Weight for a Lifetime

Weight management has two phases. If you are over-weight, losing weight is the easy part. Maintaining a healthy weight is the hard part. Think of all the people you know who have been successful at losing weight only to gain it back again. Perhaps even you?

Why do so many people have difficulty maintaining their best weight? It may be because they consider a weight control plan something they can go "on" for a period of time only to go "off" of it when they attain their goal weight. A return to old habits leads to a return to the old weight.

Lifelong weight management is about trading old habits for new ones. Specifically, it's about your eating and physical activity habits. To lose body fat and body weight, your body must burn more calories than it takes in. So if you want to lose weight or prevent weight gain, you'll need to change your eating habits *and* include more physical activity in your life.

Many people try to lose weight by simply eating less—a lot less in some cases. This causes the body's metabolism to slow down in an effort to conserve energy. You may even begin to lose some lean tissue because it is re-processed to create energy. With less lean tissue, it becomes harder to continue losing weight.

Physical activity, on the other hand, can help to keep muscle from diminishing. It also burns calories, which, coupled with eating less, can lead to a loss of body fat and, thus, weight. In fact, the single best predictor of long-term weight loss and maintenance is being physically active.

Are You Ready to Lose Weight for Good?

Losing weight is serious business. Many people tend to lose the same ten or twenty pounds over and over again. They'll lose weight for their tenth high school reunion, then for their wedding, then for a romantic Hawaii vacation, then for their twentieth high school reunion, and so on.

Research has suggested that this up and down weight change, commonly known as "yo-yo" dieting, may be harmful. Try to minimize the number of times you attempt weight loss. Try to lose weight when you are truly ready and committed to the process. Attempting weight loss when you are not ready increases your chance for failure. Failing at losing weight or keeping it off can be very demoralizing. That can negatively affect your self-esteem—not to mention your health.

Check your readiness by looking again at your responses to the "Gearing Up for Change Profile" on pages 35–37 in the "General Warranty" section. You are probably not ready to undertake a weight-loss program if you are in neutral or first gear (the precontemplation or contemplation stages) for *either* adopting a heart-healthy diet or for becoming more physically active. Why? First, as previously discussed, to lose weight successfully, you must be ready to make changes in both your diet and your activity level. Second, if you are in neutral for either area, you are probably not convinced that the advantages of adopting a heart-healthy diet or of becoming more physically active outweigh the disadvantages.

Even if you are in first gear, thinking about changing your diet or activity level is a long way from doing something about it. However, if you're in the second or third gear for *both* diet and activity, you are probably ready to begin making lasting changes in these areas—and to lose weight.

Barry is an ex-hockey player who went to work as a high school hockey and baseball coach after college. Standing on the ice with a whistle around his neck didn't burn as many calories as skating around in full pads. In fact, he had gained 25 pounds in the last few years.

When Barry had a physical exam for an insurance policy, he was told that his blood pressure was high. His doctor explained that his weight gain probably contributed to the elevated blood pressure level. So Barry started to work out after practice. He also ate only one meal a day, always at a restaurant. This was easy for him because he was a bachelor and hated to cook (mostly because he didn't know how).

Following this eating plan, Barry lost weight and fast! And his blood pressure came down with his weight. Feeling relieved that he had put his blood pressure problems behind him, Barry tapered off just a little on his activity. He also returned to eating three meals a day, usually out of a box from a restaurant. Within two months, the weight Barry had lost was back. ●

If Barry had completed the "Gearing Up for Change Profile" on pages 35–37, he probably would have found himself in the second gear for physical activity and in neutral for adopting heart-healthy eating habits. Since he wasn't ready to make permanent changes in *both* the dietary and physical activity areas, Barry just couldn't manage to keep the weight off.

Are you wondering if you're ready for permanent weight loss? Take the following quiz and find out.

READY? . . . OR NOT?

Using the scale below, indicate the degree to which each statement describes you.

> 1 = Does not describe me at all
> 2 = Describes me a little
> 3 = Describes me fairly well
> 4 = Describes me exactly

_____ I'll be satisfied with a slow rate of weight loss (one-fourth to one pound a week).

_____ I'm willing and able to make weight management a top priority in my life for the next several months.

_____ I'm willing and able to increase my physical activity level.

_____ I know that losing weight will not make my other life problems disappear.

_____ I'm willing to make changes in my diet.

_____ I feel confident in my ability to complete a self-directed weight management program.

_____ I realize that weight management is a lifelong proposition.

_____ I am committed to recording my food intake and physical activities each day.

_____ TOTAL SCORE

If your score is less than 20, you may want to delay any weight-loss attempts. Look closely at any statements on which you scored 2 or below. These may be roadblocks in your weight-loss efforts. Look at resolving these issues before attempting to lose weight now or in the future.

There may be other factors to consider before you try to lose weight. Look at the questionnaire below and see if the questions apply to you.

Other Readiness Factors to Consider		
Are you pregnant?	YES	NO
(Pregnant women should not attempt to lose weight.)		
Do you have any medical conditions that may be adversely affected by changing your eating or physical activity habits?	YES	NO
(Check with your doctor if you feel uncertain about whether or not changing your food intake and physical activity patterns would negatively affect your health.)		

Weight-Loss Skillpower

Weight management should not be taken lightly. The best advice is make your next weight-loss attempt your last. It is probably best to try to lose weight only when you are ready and when you can truly make it a priority in your life. Then it is only a matter of "skillpower" (not willpower, as many people believe). The following skills will help you prepare for and be successful with your weight-loss efforts.

TRACKING HABITS. The first step toward changing your weight is to know how your current lifestyle habits are affecting it. You can do this by developing the skill of tracking your eating and activity habits. Research shows that people who regularly monitor these habits are more likely to be successful.

Try to track for at least three days (two weekdays and one weekend day). A week or more is even better. Use the forms in Appendix A to help you monitor your daily food intake and physical activities. Remember, be accurate and honest. If you're not, the only person you'll be cheating is yourself.

Here are some tips that may help you track your food intake and your physical activity.

Food Intake Tracking Tips

- Don't change your eating habits just because you're recording the information. You want an *accurate* picture of your fat and calorie intake.
- Look up the amount of fat grams and calories you are eating. Read labels or buy a food reference book to estimate each food's fat and calorie amounts. Later you will set goals based on total fat grams and calories.
- Pay attention to people, places, feelings, or activities that tend to make you eat, especially when you are not really hungry.

Physical Activity Tracking Tips

- Write down all physical activities. From working out at the gym and walking in the neighborhood to taking the stairs at work or working in the yard—write down everything.
- Be accurate with the amount of time you actually spend moving. (Don't count rest periods between flights of stairs or sitting on a bench in the park for ten minutes.) Use a watch with a second hand or stopwatch.

Energy Summary

Use your completed food and physical activity records to fill in the information below.

My average daily calorie intake was: _____ calories

My average daily fat intake was: _____ grams

My average daily physical activity time was: _____ minutes

Kisha was always on the go. With a full-time job, a long commute, and two toddlers, she had her hands full. With all her running around, she had always figured that she was getting enough exercise. When Kisha decided that she was ready to lose some of the extra weight she had gained during her pregnancies, she kept a log of just how much physical activity she was getting each day.

As it turned out, Kisha was busy from the time she awakened to the time she went to bed (usually exhausted). But she was busy getting the kids ready for day care, driving to work, answering the phone, driving home, fixing dinner, and giving the kids their baths. Kisha had lots of activity each day, but not much of it was *physically* active.

After a close review of her log, Kisha found some places she could start adding some physical activity. At work she could climb stairs and take half of her lunch break to walk. On the weekends when she had more time, she could do something physically active. ●

SETTING GOALS. The Energy Summary on the previous page gives you an idea of your current balance between calorie intake and physical activity. Now it's time to identify where you want to go and set goals to get there.

Calorie Goals. Don't excessively restrict your calorie intake. A good place to start is to have a goal of eating 300 to 500 calories per day less than you're eating now. For example, if you found that you were averaging about 2,130 calories, you would want to keep your calorie intake to around 1,600 to 1,800 calories a day. Never restrict your calories to less than 1,200 per day.

Reducing your fat intake is important for several reasons:

- It's the most concentrated source of calories. Fat has 250 calories per ounce. Protein and carbohydrates have only 115 calories per ounce. Restricting fat will make it easier to meet your calorie goals.
- As you reduce your intake of total fat, you are likely reducing saturated fat intake as well. Studies show that saturated fat raises blood cholesterol. So a diet lower in total fat can have the added advantage of being heart-healthy.

Use the table below to determine the recommended daily fat gram intake for your weight loss calorie level. Compare this number to your current daily intake of fat grams. Chances are, you're eating more fat than is recommended for you. Use the fat

YOUR CALORIE COUNTER

Daily Weight-Loss Calorie Goal	Daily Total Fat Goal*
1200	less than 40 grams
1300	less than 43 grams
1400	less than 47 grams
1500	less than 50 grams
1600	less than 53 grams
1700	less than 57 grams
1800	less than 60 grams
1900	less than 63 grams
2000	less than 67 grams
2100	less than 70 grams
2200	less than 73 grams
2300	less than 77 grams
2400	less than 80 grams
2500	less than 83 grams
2600	less than 87 grams
2700	less than 90 grams
2800	less than 93 grams
2900	less than 97 grams
3000	less than 100 grams

*Numbers may be rounded.

gram number in the chart as your starting fat gram goal. You may find that you need to reduce this number slightly as you lose weight.

Physical Activity Goals. As a rule of thumb, gradually increase your physical activity time until you are consistently doing at least TWICE your normal amount. Remember, one easy way to increase your physical activity time is to build it into your daily activities. For example, take 15 minutes from your lunch time to walk. Start out by doing 20 percent more activity than you are now doing.

Current time × 1.2 = _____

✔ MY STARTING GOALS

Daily calorie goal: _____

Daily fat gram goal: <u>less than</u> _____ <u>grams</u>

Daily activity time goal: _____

MAKING A PLAN. Now that you have goals, it's essential that you formulate a plan to reach them. We recommend that you use a problem-solving approach like the one that follows to make your plan. For each goal area (reducing calories, reducing fat, and increasing physical activity) you should take the following steps.

1. Analyze Roadblocks. When you know your habits, you can identify your problems, the places where you need help. What information do you need? What skills are you lacking? Who can you get to help you? What are you willing to do or give up to reach your goal?

2. Specify Plans. It's time to put pencil to paper. Use the outline on the next page to guide you. Don't try to do too much at once. As you build your plan,

MY PERSONAL PLAN

1. What roadblocks do I need to overcome?

    Information to be acquired _____

    New skills to be developed _____

    People who can help _____

    What I'm willing to give up to make a change _____

2. What do I need to make the change I want?

    Name your goal (be specific and realistic): _____

    What steps will get me there?

    Start by listing your goal on the first stairstep below. Next, write on the second stairstep the last step you needed to reach your goal. Work your way down the stairsteps adding steps in reverse order, until you reach the first step—the one you can do immediately. In the blank beside each stairstep, write the date you want to achieve that step.

    ____ GOAL:_____

        ____ -_____

           ____ -_____

              ____ -_____

                 ____ -_____

                    ____ -_____

    How am I going to reward myself and those who help me? __

3. Plan on Perseverance

    There may be times when things don't work out exactly as you planned. Don't give up! Learn from your mistakes. Making changes often requires trial and error. To help keep you motivated, list the three major reasons why you want to achieve this goal:

    1. _____

    2. _____

    3. _____

4. Set aside time to review your progress and readjust your plan. I will review my plan on (list all dates):

    Write these dates in your daily calendar. Also, put your plan in a spot where you will be likely to see it regularly. Don't

forget to reward yourself when you have accomplished a goal!
For more on rewarding yourself, read pages 48–49 in the
"Operating Instructions" section under "General Warranty."

---

you may decide to break it into smaller mini-goals. It
may help to make copies of the form and use one page
for each mini-goal. Your overall plan then becomes a
collection of mini-plans.

3. Give It a Try! It's time to work your plan. Be
enthusiastic, but realize that it may take time to learn
these new skills. You may even have to adjust your
plan a little. Patience and persistence will help you be
successful. You can improve your health by losing
even a little weight. It is also an important first step to
losing more in the weeks and months ahead.

4. Review Your Plan. Periodically review your plan.
Make the adjustments necessary to stay on track or
get back on track. You may need to develop a series
of smaller goals. But don't forget to reward yourself
when you reach each goal.

RECOGNIZING HUNGER. Many things in our daily lives
trigger us to react in certain ways. (See pages 40–43 in
the "Operating Instructions" section under "General
Warranty" for more information about managing
triggers.)

Hunger is one of the most obvious eating cues. But
people who struggle with excess weight often have
difficulty knowing the difference between physiological hunger and psychological hunger. It is important
to recognize if this is a problem for you.

Physiological hunger occurs two to four hours
after your last meal. Symptoms include an empty or
rumbling feeling in your stomach, a headache, or

lightheadedness. This type of hunger is your body's way of telling you it is time to take in more food.

Psychological hunger occurs at any time and has no physical symptoms. Obsessing about food, emotional situations, certain personal triggers, or food cravings may cause you to *think* that you are hungry when you are really not.

Jay was a high school math teacher. He weighed more than he wanted to so he skipped breakfast, had only a salad at lunch, and ate a regular dinner at 6:30 p.m. Around 8:00 p.m. he usually began to feel hungry, so he raided the refrigerator for a sandwich, big bowl of ice cream, or other high-calorie snack.

After several weeks of trying to lose weight without success, Jay reevaluated his daily habits. He decided to look more closely at his 8:00 p.m. snack. On closer review he realized that the "hunger" he thought he felt was actually anxiety about preparing his lesson plans for the next day. He had been asked to teach an advanced math class, and he wasn't comfortable with the material.

Jay came up with a plan to correct the problem. First, to eliminate his feelings of anxiety, he contacted an old professor for some advice about the math class. He also decided that whenever he starts heading for the kitchen he will ask himself, "Am I really feeling hungry?" If the answer is no, he will head back to the living room, sit down, and try to figure out what triggered him to want to eat. ●

EATING LOW-FAT. When it comes to losing weight, low-fat is where it's at. As mentioned earlier, low-fat eating makes sense for a number of reasons. Counting fat grams is a skill that will help you reach your low-fat goal. But be careful. Don't forget that most low-fat and fat-free foods have calories, so you still have to watch your portion sizes. "Healthy Nutrition" on pages 57–128 of the "Service and Maintenance" section is full of strategies and techniques for reducing your fat intake.

Lupe was more than a little apprehensive about changing her diet to lose weight. All of her past weight-loss attempts had taught her that when it came to dieting, there wasn't much food she could eat and what there was didn't taste very good.

This time Lupe elected to work with Roslyn, a Registered Dietitian. They decided that a daily average of less than 45 grams of fat would be a good starting goal. Roslyn instructed Lupe on label reading and keeping logs. They talked about different strategies for reducing fat intake in cooking and how to order low-fat meals when eating out.

At the second visit two weeks later, Lupe was ecstatic. As a result of her new eating and activity habits, she had lost nearly three pounds. But what made Lupe happiest was that she never felt as if she was restricting herself. She stayed within her fat gram goal but enjoyed generous portions of vegetables, whole grains, and fruits. Never once did she feel hungry or deprived. Lupe knew that this was a "diet" she could live with for the rest of her life. ●

WHAT YOU GAIN BY BEING MORE PHYSICALLY ACTIVE. The benefits of physical activity are numerous. First, it burns calories. And when coupled with a low-fat, reduced-calorie diet, it helps you lose weight. Regular physical activity helps slow the loss of lean tissue commonly associated with weight loss and the aging process. Also, being active can improve your fitness level. Last, and perhaps most important, it can reduce your risk for heart attack and stroke.

Read "How to Keep Your Motor Humming with

Physical Activity," pages 129–210, for ways to build physical activity into your daily routine. You'll find information about starting an exercise program there as well. Remember, the key is to keep moving. Doing something is better than doing nothing.

Kevin, his wife Lori, and their three kids always went out to brunch at an all-you-can-eat steakhouse after church every Sunday. They spent the rest of the afternoon napping and sitting around trying to digest their huge meal.

Kevin recognized that this "tradition" was wreaking havoc with his waistline. So he decided to start a new tradition. On Saturday night, Kevin quickly made sandwiches, washed fruit, gathered up some low-fat tortilla chips and nonfat bean dip and tossed some fruit juice boxes into the refrigerator. He packed the nonperishables in the van and loaded all the bikes into and on top of the van.

The next morning Kevin announced that after church they were all going to the state park for a picnic and a bike ride. Excited, the kids gathered up a change of clothing while Kevin and Lori loaded the cooler into the car. Never before were the kids so eager to go to church! From then on the family shared an activity each Sunday that was physical and also a fun adventure. ●

RECOGNIZING COMMON WEIGHT-LOSS TRAPS. People do a number of things when they are trying to lose weight that put them at risk for having a setback or, worse yet, a failure. To avoid these pitfalls, keep the following tips in mind.

- Don't skip meals. Cutting out breakfast or lunch is a common way that people reduce calories.

But all it really does is set you up for an overeating episode later in the day.

- Don't weigh every day. Your weight may fluctuate from day to day due to changes in the climate, water retention, and many other factors. If you weigh every day, you may become discouraged by sudden increases in weight that are unrelated to your weight-loss efforts. Weigh no more than once a week, preferably only once a month. Record your weight on the graph in Appendix A.
- Watch out for people, programs, or products that promise a "quick fix." There are no quick fixes, just permanent changes in eating and physical activity habits.
- Don't try to lose weight from the middle of November to January first. No, there is not a climactic reason for this tip. It's the holiday season. Instead of a weight-loss goal, set a goal to not gain any weight during the holidays. That is goal enough.
- Watch out for distorted thinking. Such thinking can trigger a lapse. For example:

    All or Nothing Thinking. "I can't do more than ten minutes of my workout today, so I might as well skip the whole thing."

    Perfectionistic Thinking. "I've started eating low-fat food today. That means bye-bye chocolate forever."

- Resist "testing" yourself once you've lost some weight. It's common for people who successfully lost weight to cut back on their activity or go back to eating the foods that were particularly troublesome for them. They do it just to see if they can get away with it.
- Be mindful of negative feelings or moods. Your self control disappears if you are depressed, anx-

ious, stressed out, or simply frustrated for a prolonged period. Find ways to cope with these feelings.

Getting support for your efforts, managing triggers, and preventing relapses are just some of the strategies discussed in detail in Chapter Three titled "How to Keep Your Heart Finely Tuned," beginning on page 30. Review these ideas and choose the ones that will work best for you. Remember, losing weight and keeping it off is not about willpower—it's all about *skill*power.

Evaluating a Weight Control Program

When evaluating and selecting a weight control book or program, make sure it meets the following criteria.

• *It Is Nutritionally Adequate.* The diet plan should be well-balanced and should include a variety of low-fat foods.

• *It Emphasizes Physical Activity.* Regular physical activity is one of the strongest predictors of long-term weight management success.

• *It Meets Dietary Guidelines.* The total fat, saturated fat, cholesterol, and sodium content of the recommended diet plan should be in line with the current recommendations of the American Heart Association.

• *It Evaluates Readiness.* The psychological and perhaps physical consequences of "on again, off again" dieting can be severe. Only committed and motivated people should attempt weight loss.

• *It Supports a Slow Weight Loss.* Gradual changes in eating, activity, and thinking habits allow you to adjust better to new habits and skills. Your likelihood of failure is high if you go on a "crash" diet. Don't expect more than a one-quarter to one pound weight loss per week.

• *It Helps You Learn Change Skills.* Monitoring

your food intake and daily activity are important skills. So are coping with triggers, giving yourself rewards, and preparing for setbacks.

• *It Fits Your Lifestyle.* If you have to drastically change your daily routine or activities, you might not be able to stick to the program.

 Weight-Loss Facts and Fallacies

If a weight-loss book is on the bestseller list, it must really work, right?

Not necessarily. No one regulates diet books in the same way that the federal government regulates food labels. That means that an author can put virtually anything into a book, whether or not it is scientifically proven. "Quack" diet books may become bestsellers because of gimmicks that make their diet plan seem new, innovative, and different from all others. The gimmick may be the way the author suggests eating foods in specified combinations. Or the book may tout the "magical" qualities of a certain food or food group. One common gimmick is to condemn a particular food group (such as milk) and leave it out of the diet entirely. Always the author says his or her diet plan is "easy," "painless," and of course, "effective."

With a flashy cover, an intense marketing campaign, and a nationwide book tour, many such books become instant bestsellers. How do these books stay on the bestseller list for months, even years? Say you bought one of the books. You followed the diet plan and lost eight pounds in two weeks. (It's mostly water loss, but the authors don't tell you that.) All your friends and family are so impressed, they want to know how you did it. You give them the book title and they make a mad dash to the store.

After another two weeks your friends and family are getting "results" too. Their friends want to know how, and they, too, go buy a copy. Meanwhile, you are four weeks into the program and you have given up. You have gained back most of the weight you lost in the beginning and can't stick to the restrictive diet any longer.

Since there is never a money-back guarantee on these kinds of books, you have no other option but to throw the book in the trash. More than likely, you'll blame yourself for failing. All the while, people are spreading the word (at least for the first two weeks) about this amazing new diet plan! Soon it's a bestseller with nothing to offer but nutrition misinformation and scientific half-truths.

Is it true that unused muscle becomes fat?

No. The body does not convert muscle tissue to fat. What gives this impression is that unused muscle tissue shrinks a little. If body fat is added, it lies over the muscle just under the skin, giving the appearance that the muscle has turned to fat.

I want to lose a lot of fat off my buttocks and thighs. Will stair climbing accomplish this goal?

Yes and no. Stair climbing is a vigorous activity that burns a lot of calories. This, coupled with a low-fat diet, can contribute to fat loss. But you can't lose fat at one site and not at others. Stair climbing will simply strengthen and tone the muscles in these areas, which may give the appearance that weight loss has occurred.

HIGHLIGHTS ─────────────────────────

Losing Weight, Gaining Health

When you can maintain your best weight, you'll be doing your heart and blood vessels a big favor. But don't try to do it all overnight. And remember, don't be misled by fad diets.

CHAPTER EIGHT

Preventing Breakdowns and Blow-ups

 Keeping Everyday Stress Under Control

Driving in excessive heat or at extremely high speeds can really stress your car. This is especially true if it's not in good condition. Low oil pressure, inadequate radiator fluid, or transmission problems can make stressful driving conditions even harder on your car—and potentially damaging.

Humans are the same way. Traffic jams, deadlines, financial difficulties, relationship problems, and hectic schedules are just a few examples of the many stressful situations in our lives. Studies show that the way we respond to these situations and events may affect our health, including our risk of heart attack and stroke.

The good news is that we can protect our health by coping with the factors that stress us. This chapter describes how stress management, relaxation techniques, communication skills, and self-esteem can

258

protect us from both the short- and long-term hazards associated with stress.

Emotional Health and Your Heart

In the 1950's the term "Type-A Personality" was first used to describe a number of behavioral tendencies observed in many heart patients. These Type-A tendencies were competitiveness, driving ambition, impatience, hostility, and time urgency (always in a hurry to accomplish more in less time). In contrast, people who didn't exhibit these traits were described as having "Type-B" personalities.

Numerous research studies have since investigated and supported the connection between the Type-A Personality and heart disease. They found that Type-A individuals developed heart disease at 2 to 2.2 times the rate of Type-B's. They found this to be the case even when taking into consideration other risk factors such as smoking, family history of heart disease, high blood pressure, and obesity. Type-A personalities also had an increased risk of developing angina pectoris, chest pain associated with physical exertion.

In the years that followed, the term "Type-A Personality" was replaced by the term "Coronary-Prone Behavior Pattern" (CPBP). This suggested a cluster of *behaviors* rather than a global personality. It also allowed researchers to examine each aspect of the behavior pattern to determine which behaviors were the most unhealthy. Since a specific behavior is more easily changed than an entire personality, this shift in terminology reflected the hope that people could change unhealthy behaviors.

Additional research showed that not all aspects of the Coronary-Prone Behavior Pattern were equally unhealthy. Ambition, impatience, time-urgency, competitiveness, and strong work and achievement drives were not found to predict heart disease. But in study after study, one behavior *did* correlate with heart disease: anger and hostility.

To fully understand the relationship between hostility and coronary artery disease, it's important to look at the three distinct aspects of hostility.

- *Hostility* is a chronic attitude or way of looking at the world. It involves cynical mistrust of others, suspiciousness, resentment, and self-centeredness.
- *Anger* is an episodic emotion or feeling that may range from mild annoyance or irritation to rage.
- *Aggression* is the behavioral expression of anger, either through verbal or physical threat (yelling, cursing, hitting).

Steve hated to go to the grocery store because he thought that everyone he saw there was an "idiot." The butcher was lazy when he failed to respond to the first ring of the bell. The deli-man purposely sliced his ham too thickly, just because Steve told him he didn't have all day. And the check-out person was obviously an airhead who was more interested in chatting with other customers in the line ahead of him than in doing her job.

And why couldn't those people on aisle three control those bratty kids who kept screaming? He began to mutter obscenities under his breath when people in front of him had coupons or could not find their checkbooks. The last straw came when he noticed the jerk in the express line ahead of him with eighteen items instead of fifteen. Feeling thoroughly infuriated, Steve loudly berated the offender and told him to go get in another line. ●

In the story above, Steve's hostile attitude is illustrated by his tendency to perceive others as stupid, lazy, incompetent, and rude. Feelings of anger began with annoyance at the butcher and escalated to rage at the check-out line. Aggressive behavior was expressed through muttering obscenities, being sarcastic with the deli manager, and screaming at the other customer in line.

Anger itself is not necessarily a "bad" emotion. Anger helps us set boundaries with others and protect ourselves. It's only a problem if it occurs too often or easily, or if it is expressed inappropriately.

On the down side, the emotion that comes with anger causes stress hormones to be released into the bloodstream. This may increase blood pressure, heart and breathing rates, and muscle tension. It may also slow digestion. Some scientists call these "anger chemicals." Studies have suggested that they affect the body's arteries, constricting and dilating them as blood is circulated to the large muscle groups. These chemicals are thought to prepare the body for two possible self-protection options: to fight or to run.

Some scientists believe that anger is most harmful when "bottled up" or suppressed—so called "anger-in." Several studies compared groups of "anger-in" people with groups of people who vent or express anger ("anger-out"). They found that high blood pressure is more common among "anger-in" individuals. The study also found a higher heart attack risk in "anger-in" groups. Researchers disagree on this point. Some believe that people who openly express their anger have more health problems.

Most agree, however, that the most healthful approach involves "cool reflection." Healthy anger is not chronic, and it is expressed assertively and appropriately toward the correct target. Unhealthy anger is chronic anger that occurs regularly and is expressed inappropriately, indirectly, suppressed, or acted out aggressively.

Among men whose blood pressure was monitored, the lowest blood pressure was found in those who acknowledged their anger but were not openly aggressive or hostile. Highest blood pressures were found in those with either "bottled-up" anger or openly hostile behavior. Openly hostile behavior frequently results in making the situation worse or in harming relationships.

Hostile people become angry more often and with greater intensity than other people. One study indicated that hostility affects the body much like stress. Since hostility is chronic, it can appear to create a fairly frequent or constant release of stress hormones. This increases blood pressure and heart rate, and it stimulates the liver to release cholesterol and triglycerides into the blood.

Hostility may also cause increased testosterone levels. High testosterone levels may contribute to lowering HDL levels (the "good" cholesterol). In one study, 830 people were tested for hostility in college and followed up twenty years later. Those with high hostility in college had higher total blood cholesterol and lower levels of HDL.

One study assessed the hostility levels of 400 people about to undergo a coronary arteriography. (This is a medical procedure that looks at the flow of blood in the arteries feeding the heart.) The study found that 70 percent of the hostile patients had at least one major blockage of a coronary artery. Only 48 percent of the non-hostile group had such blockage. Hostile patients were 1.5 times more likely to have blockages than non-hostile patients.

Many researchers believe that there is a correlation between hostility and disease. Hostility seems to have direct harmful physical effects on the body. Furthermore, hostile people tend to drive others away. This may make the correlation even stronger.

One Swedish study reported that hostile people who were socially isolated had three times the death rate from heart disease than people with a strong support group. Numerous studies during the past decade have similarly demonstrated that social support is a powerful buffer against illness.

Aside from the inappropriate expression of anger, another aspect of hostility that may decrease social support is the tendency of hostile people to be self-centered. A self-centered person can perceive any event as a personal threat: other drivers are seen as intentionally rude; lane changes are viewed as hostile intrusions into one's personal space.

One study found that people who used more self-references in their speech (I, me, my) had higher blood pressure during stressful tasks. Taped conversations of people's discussions have shown that excessive self-referencing (I, me, my) correlated with disease severity and predicted heart problems. Self-referencing and hostility are related in that if one is hostile toward others, he is also likely to be more self-involved.

 ## Stress Management: Taking a New Look at Your Assumptions

It's popular to think that stress is something that occurs outside of yourself. For example, you may think to yourself, "I feel stressed out because this traffic is a mess and I'm going to be late for my appointment." But in fact, stress is your reaction to this event—it happens inside you. The symptoms of acute stress include mental alertness and emotional reactions such as fear or anger. Stress may also cause a temporary increase in heart rate and blood pressure.

A certain amount of stress is healthy. It helps us feel challenged and energized. Healthy stress, called "eustress," keeps us from feeling bored and provides a sense of purpose in life. But too much stress, called "distress," can be extremely harmful to our relationships, health, and emotional well-being. This is especially true when it occurs repeatedly or over a long period of time. That's why it's critical to manage the stress in your life, even though it may not always be easy. Start by taking it one step at a time, using the following steps designed to help you manage stress.

STEP ONE: RECOGNIZING THE STRESS. The first step in managing unhealthy stress is to learn to recognize the early warning signals. By doing that, you can start appropriate coping measures before your health and well-being are threatened. These early warning signals may be:

- physical, such as muscle tension, upset stomach, or fatigue;
- mental, such as worry, confusion, or distractibility;
- emotional, such as irritability, anxiety, or a temporarily depressed mood; and,
- behavioral, such as temper outbursts, accident proneness, social withdrawal, or substance abuse.

Each person experiences different warning signals of stress. It's important to become aware of yours so that you can interrupt the stress cycle as soon as it starts. Otherwise, stress builds over time as negative, unhealthy coping begins to make the original problem even worse.

● Bob started worrying when multiple layoffs occurred at work. He worked longer hours in an
attempt to avoid losing his job. Bob believed that "real
men" shouldn't admit either to themselves or to others
that they were "stressed out." He considered it a sign
of weakness. As a result, he became more preoccupied, withdrawn, and irritable at home. To escape the
pressure and relax, Bob began to drink more. His
drinking only increased his tendency to withdraw and
lash out at others. His wife, Sandy, tried repeatedly to
reach out to Bob, without success. After several
months, Sandy initiated a trial separation. This created
yet another source of stress for Bob.

As he became more depressed over the state of his
marriage, Bob experienced sleep difficulties, which
hurt his job performance. The next round of layoffs
found Bob's name at the top of the list. ●

Let's assume that Bob had recognized his early
warning signs of distress rather than denying them and
masking them with alcohol. When he noticed and
admitted that his anxiety, withdrawal, preoccupation,
and moodiness were signs of stress, he could have
taken the next important step in managing his stress.
That is accepting responsibility for managing his response to the situation.

STEP TWO: ACCEPTING RESPONSIBILITY FOR YOUR RE-
SPONSE. Accepting responsibility for your own stress
response empowers you to deal with the source of the
stress as well as your feelings about it. Accepting
responsibility doesn't mean blaming yourself for feeling stressed. Rather, it means that you agree it's up to
you to manage the impact of stress on both yourself
and your relationships.

STEP THREE: LOOK FOR THE SOURCE OF YOUR STRESS.
The next step is to look for the source of stress, called
the stressor. A stressor may be an event outside
yourself, such as being the victim of a crime. Or it can
originate within yourself, such as if you were to imagine
something terrible happening to someone you love.

In the 1960's, researchers thought that stress was
caused by major life events like marriage, divorce, or
job loss. They developed life event scales to measure
how much stress people experience in those situations. More recently, researchers have shifted their
focus from these infrequent major life events to the
ongoing stresses and strains of everyday living, which
they labeled "hassles."

Although less traumatic than major life events,
everyday hassles may be more dangerous because
they occur more frequently, in fact, continuously. For
example, hassles would include such everyday events
as losing things, not having enough time, commuting
in traffic, and friction with a co-worker, boss, or
spouse.

A major life event may result in numerous daily
hassles. For example, divorce may result in having to
learn new tasks, juggle finances, adjust your recreational activities, raise your spouse's children, seek
out new friends, or find a new place to live. Hassles
provide a "double whammy" because they seem so
trivial that you are often not aware of how seriously
they affect you. At the same time, others may not
recognize that you are stressed out and need help.

Some people don't need major life events or hassles to create stress for themselves. Chronic worriers
create their own stress internally by focusing on terrible events that may never occur. You've heard it
before: "I dented that guy's fender. *What if* he sues
me for neck injuries?" or "My child is 20 minutes
late. *What if* she's been killed in a car accident?"

Unfortunately for these people, *"what if"* thinking produces the same stress response in our bodies as actual stressful events.

When you've identified a stressor, try to determine to what extent it's within your ability to control. People often waste valuable time and energy trying to correct or "fix" a situation that is simply outside of their control. On the other hand, if anything can be done to improve the situation, take steps to deal with it. If chronic marital conflict is stressing you out, for example, solutions might include:

- talking out your problems with your spouse and attempting to negotiate;
- seeing a marriage counselor;
- resolving to behave differently toward your partner; or
- getting a divorce.

STEP FOUR: EXAMINE YOUR BELIEFS AND ATTITUDES. Is your own thinking adding to your distress? The life event scale had one major drawback. It didn't explain why some people with many life events did not become ill, while others with few events did. This suggested that stress is much more complicated than merely what happens to you. Researchers concluded that, "stress is in the eye of the beholder." In other words, you must think something is stressful for it to be so. No matter what it is, if you don't think it's stressful, it won't be.

John traveled a lot for his job and became so accustomed to flying that he totally "tuned out." He became so involved in reading the newspaper that he had no idea when the plane took off or hit mild turbulence. Robert, on the other hand, really enjoyed opportunities for air travel. He always asked for a window seat and loved to watch the takeoffs and landings, as well as any scenery visible below. He found the sounds and movements of the plane so relaxing that they frequently lulled him to sleep.

In contrast, Tom dreaded flying because he always felt anxious and nervous. He envisioned fiery crashes as he recalled in vivid detail news stories of multiple fatalities in last year's air disaster. He focused on each sound of the engines or any movement of the plane, fearing that each signaled serious mechanical trouble. As he tightly clutched the armrest, he felt his heart pounding. By the time he reached his destination, he had a terrible headache. ●

The same event—an airplane ride—can be neutral to some people (as in John's case); exciting and interesting to others (as in Robert's case); or highly upsetting and stressful (as in Tom's case). In fact, the event itself was neutral, but each person's thoughts about the event determined its stressfulness.

This is important to know for several reasons. First, remember that your body responds to your thoughts, beliefs, and images as if they were *real* events. So, even though nothing out of the ordinary was happening during the flight, Tom's body reacted. He had a full-blown stress response as if his life were threatened—simply because that's how he thought about it.

This means that much of your stress load is under your own control. While you can't always control external events, you can work to control how you think and feel about them.

Behaviorists have identified certain thinking patterns that almost always create stress, not only for the person thinking them, but also for people around them. Three specific beliefs tend to create significant stress:

- the need for approval,
- perfectionistic thinking, and
- low frustration tolerance.

The *need for approval* could be expressed as, "I must have the approval and acceptance of almost everyone I meet, and if I don't, I'm a worthless, no-good person." Approval seekers have difficulty saying no, setting appropriate limits, and expressing their own needs. Since it's impossible to please everyone, no matter how much one tries, approval seekers frequently experience feelings of rejection where none is intended.

Perfectionistic thinking could be expressed as, "I must not make errors or do poorly, and if I do, it's terrible." This thought is irrational since no human being is perfect and everyone makes mistakes. By setting impossible standards, the perfectionist dooms himself to feeling like a perpetual failure.

Low frustration tolerance could be expressed as, "People and events must (or should) conform to my desires and wishes, and if they don't, I can't stand it." People with low frustration tolerance have a mental list of shoulds, musts, and oughts. They apply these to the world and others as a set of rules that should be followed. Examples of these beliefs include people should drive a certain way, should be on time, shouldn't litter, or should remember your birthday. People with these rigid expectations create chronic stress for themselves and others, since other people's internal rules rarely match their own.

STEP FIVE: EMPLOY STRESS REDUCTION TECHNIQUES AND ACTIVITIES. Try to reduce or discharge your bodily stress using stress reduction techniques or activities. These might include:

- talking to a good friend about the problem,

- exercising,
- doing a relaxation technique,
- getting a massage,
- taking a warm bath,
- meditating,
- engaging in a physically demanding hobby, or
- seeking out a funny movie or other laughter-producing event.

Take a moment now to list activities that you find helpful in discharging stress and tension.

- _____
- _____
- _____
- _____
- _____

 ## Relaxation Techniques: A Health-Giving Lift

Fortunately, there is a potent and natural antidote to stress that does not involve alcohol or other drugs. It's called the relaxation response. This response is the complete opposite of the stress response. It's also associated with decreased heart rate and blood pressure, relaxed muscles, slower breathing, slower brain waves, and a return to a low level of stress.

The relaxation response can help you cope with stress in two ways. First, when practiced for 15 to 20 minutes a day on a regular basis, it can help reduce your overall stress level and improve your health. Studies have shown that regular relaxation practice results in better immune function and lowered blood cholesterol. Second, when you learn this skill well, you can use brief relaxation techniques repeatedly during the day to help reduce stress whenever you feel it. For example, after nearly having an accident on the freeway, a well-practiced individual can immediately reverse the stress response, lowering it to a safe level. This is much better than letting it build up along with other stressors as the day progresses.

People relax in different ways. They may work in the garden, watch television, play golf, read, or go to the movies. But these types of activities may not result in the same deep levels of relaxation that can be achieved by the relaxation techniques described below. In fact, you can obtain a deep level of relaxation through:

- meditation,
- progressive muscle relaxation,
- visualization or imaging, and
- diaphragmatic breathing.

MEDITATION. One of these techniques is meditation. To try it, just follow this simple, step-by-step outline.

1. Pick a word, phrase, image, or suggestion to focus on. The mental focus could be neutral, such as "one"; suggestive, such as "calm"; or even a prayerful meditative phrase, such as "peace, love, or joy."
2. Sit quietly in a comfortable position.
3. Close your eyes.
4. Relax your muscles.
5. Breathe slowly and dwell on your mental focus by repeating it over and over.
6. Assume a passive attitude, particularly with regard to intrusive thoughts or how well you are doing.
7. Continue for ten to twenty minutes.
8. Practice once or twice daily.

PROGRESSIVE MUSCLE RELAXATION. This technique involves systematically tensing, and then relaxing, various muscle groups in your body. With continued practice over time, you will begin to learn to recognize and reduce even subtle muscle tension that accompanies stress. An abbreviated version of this technique follows.

Since it's common to hold your breath when tense, remember to breathe throughout the entire tension-relaxation cycle. Close your eyes and tense each muscle group listed below one at a time in the order given, to about 50 percent maximum tenseness. Hold the tension for a few seconds as you continue to breathe, then release the tension. Pause and tune into your body after each relaxation phase, noticing the difference between tension and relaxation in your body.

1. Neck and shoulders—tense, pause, release tension, notice the contrast.
2. Face—tense, pause, release tension, study the difference.
3. Hands and arms—tense, pause, release tension, study the contrast.
4. Buttocks and thighs—tense, pause, release tension, tune into your body.
5. Calves and feet—tense, pause, release tension, become aware of the contrast.

Sit quietly and enjoy the feeling of deep relaxation for several minutes before counting backward from ten to one as you slowly return to full alertness.

VISUALIZATION—MAKING RELAXATION A HABIT. Visualization or imaging involves sitting quietly, closing your eyes, and imagining yourself in a peaceful, relaxing scene. This scene may be an especially vivid memory of a wonderful place you have actually seen or visited. In a guided visualization, someone else suggests a peaceful image to you. If any suggested image has a negative association for you, it is important to switch to another, more relaxing image. The following abbreviated example illustrates this technique.

Imagine you are walking down a beautiful sandy beach at the edge of the ocean. The clear, crystal blue water washes over your feet as you walk. The sand feels soft and cool beneath your feet and between your toes. Your shoulder muscles begin to relax as they absorb the soothing warmth of the sun. You feel a gentle, cool ocean breeze against your face and arms. You decide to sit down and absorb the beauty around you. Leaving your feet in the water, you slowly lean back on your hands and feel the warm sand beneath your hands. You begin to dig your fingers and hands slowly into the sand and the warmth envelops your hands and fingers.

Closing your eyes, you hear the rhythmic ocean waves breaking as they approach the shore. You become aware of seagulls calling out as they glide across the sky. Their repetitive cries lull you into deeper and deeper relaxation.

You feel peaceful, safe, and close to nature. Enjoy that peaceful feeling for several more minutes before slowly opening your eyes and returning to your current time and place. ●

DIAPHRAGMATIC OR DEEP ABDOMINAL BREATHING. When stressed, people tend to breathe rapidly and shallowly. Also, tight clothing and attempts to hold in the stomach combine to force breathing movements away from the diaphragm, the primary breathing muscle, and upward into the chest and shoulders. This shift results in shallow breathing called thoracic, reversed, or chest breathing.

Shallow breathing can be seen in hyperventilation

syndrome, which is often associated with panic attacks. Training in deep diaphragmatic breathing aims to return the breathing to a slow, natural, rhythmic pattern. The following example illustrates only one of several different ways to accomplish abdominal breathing.

Sit quietly in an upright, comfortable position and close your eyes. Place your right hand on your chest and your left hand on your abdomen. Mentally count slowly from one to four as you inhale and pause briefly at the top of the breath. Then slowly count from one to six as you exhale. Count at your own comfortable pace. Notice which hand moves as you breathe. Try to slowly shift most of the movement toward your lower hand. Feel your lower hand rise as you inhale, and fall as you exhale.

Continue to breathe and count as you observe the movements of your lower hand. After several minutes of breathing slowly and rhythmically, open your eyes and sit quietly. Enjoy the feeling of peacefulness that accompanies deep, slow breathing. ●

Once mastered, deep abdominal breathing is an excellent technique that can be used anytime, anyplace to reduce stress. It can be done with eyes open in a meeting, before a stressful event such as public speaking or a job interview, or to recover from an unpleasant interaction or conflict. In time, diaphragmatic breathing may once again become your habitual breathing pattern, just as it was when you were an infant.

PRACTICE TIPS. In the early stages of learning relaxation techniques, it is important not to practice them when you are extremely tired, upset, or angry. It is too difficult to learn a new skill under negative circumstances. For example, imagine trying to learn to ride a bicycle on a very rocky, uneven terrain. Although impossible for a novice, a very experienced bike rider could negotiate such a trail with little difficulty. In the same way, after you learn relaxation techniques through consistent practice, you can eventually use them as valuable coping tools in even the most stressful situations.

The relaxation response is helpful in relieving headaches, reducing angina pain, lowering blood pressure and cholesterol, alleviating insomnia, anxiety, and stress. Of course, it's not a substitute for good medical care. It's simply considered an adjunct to it. The regular, consistent practice of these techniques may alter your physical functioning. If you have a chronic medical condition requiring daily medication, tell your doctor so that appropriate medical follow-up and medication management can be done.

 Focus on Your Communication Skills

Communication is a "two-way street." It requires both a "sender" and a "receiver." People who truly communicate realize that listening is every bit as important as talking.

ACTIVE LISTENING. Active listening is a technique that helps the receiver avoid jumping to conclusions, mind reading, becoming defensive, or making too rapid a response. Active listening sends a powerful message to the speaker that he is being heard and respected. Here's how it works.

As the listener, you sit quietly without interrupting the speaker until he or she has stopped talking. Make eye contact with the speaker and do nothing else but

276   Your Heart: *An Owner's Manual*

listen. When the speaker stops talking, reflect back to the speaker the basic message you believe that you heard. You may also want to reflect back any feelings that you heard in the message. Then ask the speaker if your understanding of the message was accurate, and *wait for a response.* Ask for any additional information or details you need in order to fully understand the message.

Thirteen-year-old Johnny burst in the door, slammed his books on the table, and said to his mother, "I hate school! I wish I could drop out!"

Working absently in the kitchen, his mother said, "Oh, you don't mean that. You know how important a good education is."

"Yes I do mean it!" Johnny screamed. "They're all a bunch of stupid jerks!"

"Well, you don't sound so mature yourself right now. Just go to your room if you're going to act like a two-year-old."

"You just don't understand!" Johnny said as he stomped out of the room crying. ●

Compare the above scenario to the same situation in which the mother uses active listening.

Thirteen-year-old Johnny burst in the door, slammed his books on the table, and said, "I hate school! I wish I could drop out!"

Working absently in the kitchen, his mother stopped what she was doing and turned to Johnny. "Sounds like you're really upset about something that happened at school today, and you wish you didn't even have to be there."

"That's right," Johnny replied. "The other guys tease me because I'm so short. I guess I'll never start growing!"

"The guys were teasing you about your height. Does that make you begin to worry about it?"

"I do that anyway—I don't need them to remind me of it."

"You've been worrying about your height for a while, haven't you?"

"Yeah, do you think I'll *ever* grow up?" ●

Notice how the mother's unwillingness to listen in the first scenario only served to reinforce Johnny's questioning of his maturity. The communication stopped abruptly with both parties feeling disturbed and upset. In contrast, his mother's active listening in the second scenario encouraged Johnny to open up about his *real* concerns. This stimulated a discussion of an extremely important topic in this young man's life.

PROCESSING THE INFORMATION. After you've received the message, the next step is to process the information. Too often, people respond impulsively to someone else before checking out their own assumptions or thinking things through. It's important to delay your response, if necessary, in order to calm down or collect your thoughts. This also gives you time to ask for additional information and clarification. It allows you to remain emotionally calm and detached from the content of the message. That way, you're more likely to focus on the message itself, rather than to go off on a tangent or react defensively.

RESPONDING TO THE INFORMATION. After receiving and processing the message the next step is to reply, which involves both verbal and non-verbal signals. Some of these methods of replying are appropriate; others are not.

Passive Replies. When a passive person replies, he or she often does not speak up, express feelings, or ask for what he or she wants. A passive person's body language might include poor eye contact, head being turned down or away, words mumbled, quiet or muted voice, body "closed" (arms folded, shoulders hunched).

With this communication style, a passive person's thoughts and feelings cannot be known by others. As a result, they may be taken for granted or exploited. In addition, passive people usually have increased stress because they fail to set limits and get their needs met. They internalize their anger, and let their feelings build up, becoming chronic over time. As a result, passive individuals often feel resentful, angry, depressed, fearful, and anxious.

Aggressive Replies. The verbal behavior of aggressive people may include attacking, threatening, blaming, demanding, name calling, putting others down, and cursing. Body language is characterized by a loud voice and explosive speech. Gestures may be threatening such as a finger pointing and a fist pounding. Facial expressions might include scowling and frowning. They may also invade the body space of other people ("in your face"). In extreme cases, they may become physically aggressive.

The natural result of one person's aggressive behavior is that other people often become defensive, frightened, or angry. These strong feelings then interfere with their ability or willingness to listen to the angry person. Aggressive people are less likely to get what they want from the interaction. They may lose social support, damage relationships, and become isolated. The aggressive person will feel anger, frustration, and rage.

Passive-Aggressive Replies. Passive-aggressive individuals express anger and aggression in indirect ways so that other people cannot defend themselves. If confronted by others about their inappropriate behavior, passive-aggressive people deny that they meant anything by it and question why others are "so defensive."

Passive-aggressive verbal behaviors include sarcasm, inappropriate use of humor, or muttering under one's breath. Passive-aggressive behaviors include procrastination, chronic lateness, frequent forgetting, and losing of others' possessions. Passive-aggressive non-verbal behaviors include facial expressions such as smirking and rolling the eyes, sulking, and withdrawing. Passive-aggressive people make other people feel angry, full of rage, frustrated, and confused. Although passive-aggressive behavior may seem to work for these people in the short term, it eventually "boomerangs." That's because others eventually learn to avoid them, resulting in social isolation and rejection.

Assertive Replies. The healthiest way to communicate is through assertive behavior, the honest and direct expression of your thoughts, needs, and feelings. The first step in becoming assertive is to believe that you have certain basic personal rights. These include the right to express your opinion, to ask for what you want, to express your feelings honestly, to say "no," to ask questions, and to set limits and boundaries with others.

The second assertiveness skill is the ability to remain emotionally calm and sufficiently detached. This will allow you to express yourself appropriately and to avoid an unnecessary and escalating conflict.

Third, learn how to express yourself clearly, honestly, and forthrightly. Develop a strong posture with an "open" body stance. This means that your shoulders are squared, your head is up and facing the listener, and your arms are free to move. You also need good eye contact, a strong firm voice, and clearly enunciated speech.

Although assertive behavior does not guarantee that you will always get what you want, it significantly increases the odds that you will. Assertive behavior decreases stress because you are more likely to get your needs met, express your feelings appropriately, and set limits with others. An assertive person is likely to feel calm and confident, and is more likely to have good relationships and strong social support.

To increase healthy communication through assertiveness, write down and memorize your list of personal rights. Repeat this list firmly several times a day. To develop the calm detachment necessary for clear assertive communication, practice relaxation techniques such as deep breathing and muscle relaxation. After relaxing to remain calm, listen actively, and ask for clarifying information.

It is often helpful to delay your response to a confrontation. A delay of several seconds to several days may give you time to calm down, gather your thoughts, and formulate an appropriate reply. This delay can be accomplished by saying, "I hear what you are saying. Let me take a second to think about it," or "This is really important. Let me think about it and get back to you later."

Communicate with "I" statements rather than "you" statements, which tend to be blaming and demanding. Take a look at these two examples. "I get really nervous when you drive this fast. Would you please slow down?" This is more likely to get a cooperative response than the following alternative. "You're driving way too fast. Why are you always in such a hurry?"

An assertive person aims for a "win-win" resolution, by negotiating or compromising if necessary. Any communication in which your goal is to win at the expense of another person will be disappointing. While you may, in fact, win the battle, you will lose the war if the other person ends up feeling humiliated or resentful.

To improve your non-verbal communication skills, rehearse scenarios in front of a mirror and on audio tape. Listen to your voice quality and observe your body language. Before a job interview or a confrontation with your spouse, visualize the situation and "rehearse" the appropriate assertive behaviors.

To improve your general assertiveness skills, ask an assertive friend to role play different situations with you and give you honest feedback about your behavior. Practice some of the following situations: saying "no" to a request; asking for a favor; disagreeing with an opinion; or responding to a confrontation.

Finally, an extremely important but frequently overlooked aspect of effective communication is timing. People often make the mistake of bringing up "touchy" subjects at the wrong time. This may be when the other person is watching television, reading a book, stressed out, or tired. It works best to first ask the other person what time would be convenient to have a discussion about something important to you. Then set an appointment if necessary.

 ## Self-Esteem: Secret of Emotional Health

Self-esteem typically refers to how we *value* ourselves as people—whether we view ourselves as basically good. In contrast to this is self-concept, which is how we *see* ourselves.

For example, self-concept would include beliefs

such as "I am smart," "I am not artistically talented," "I am assertive," or "I am shy." Self-esteem is based on how we value or judge such traits or behaviors. That's why people can realistically describe their traits in a positive way, yet still report having feelings of worthlessness.

Self-esteem begins in early childhood and may derive from messages we receive from parents, teachers, friends, and others. The degree of love and acceptance around us during these formative years builds a foundation for later feelings toward ourselves. In addition, self-esteem may be influenced by physical limitations, appearance, social class, and how well we do in school. Self-esteem can also be influenced by how we talk to ourselves in adulthood.

Sarah arrived at the gym to watch her husband play racquetball. As the game progressed, she watched with growing irritation as the other player repeatedly screamed insults every time her husband made an especially good shot. The man yelled, "You idiot," "You stupid jerk," and other angry put-downs throughout the game. Her husband completely ignored the man and continued to increase his lead.

When the match was finally over, Sarah congratulated her husband on his win. She also remarked that she didn't know how he could so calmly tolerate the other player's hostile abuse.

"Oh, he wasn't screaming at *me*," he said. "He was mad at himself!" ●

Most people would never talk to a child in such an abusive way. In fact, child-rearing experts emphasize the importance of parents giving unconditional love to their children. Parents are told, "Never criticize the *child*; criticize the *behavior*." Most parents now understand the importance of "separating the child from his behavior." For example, "Billy, I won't tolerate your lying to me" focuses on the behavior. It is preferable to "Billy, you're a little liar" or, even worse, "Billy, you're a bad boy."

Even though we have become sensitive to these issues in children, many adults fail to apply these same principles to themselves. We apply rigid expectations and demands, expect perfection, and think in terms of global labels. We often make our self-approval and feelings of self-worth dependent on external achievements. Instead, it's important to accept ourselves unconditionally despite our human shortcomings.

Ted told his therapist that he had developed very poor self-esteem and feelings of worthlessness over the past year. He explained he was a failure at work when just the year before he had been the star sales representative. The worst thing about it, he said, was that the sales representatives were rank-ordered by sales volume. The results for the year were publicly posted on the company bulletin board, which he found extremely humiliating.

Thinking that Ted's performance at work must have plummeted during the past year, the therapist asked how many sales representatives worked for the company.

"Sixteen," he replied.

"Were you near the bottom of the list?"

"No, I was number two."

"Why is that a problem?" she asked.

"Well, if I'm not number one, then as far as I'm concerned, I'm a failure." ●

Ted's first mistake was to base his feelings of self-worth on external performance. His second mistake was judging his worthiness as a human being by comparing himself to others. Basing your self-esteem on anything outside yourself is dangerous for two reasons. First, no one's performance can always be outstanding. Second, no matter what criteria we base our self-esteem on, someone will almost certainly eventually do better than we can.

An Olympic gymnast is injured and cannot compete. A concert pianist loses concentration and fails to win the competition. A star football player runs the wrong way with the ball. What do these people have in common? All will feel like miserable failures if their self-esteem is based solely on external achievement.

In addition to causing psychological difficulties, poor self-esteem can also affect your physical health. People who feel worthless are less likely to take good care of themselves. They are likely to be less assertive and, therefore, will be subject to more stress. One study looked at people with low self-esteem. When involved in stressful, problem-solving tasks, these people showed more hostility than did high self-esteem subjects. As noted earlier, hostility is strongly implicated as a risk factor for cardiovascular disease.

In order to escape the trap of poor self-esteem, you must give up the idea of pursuing high self-esteem. If you feel great about yourself today because you won a contest, you will almost certainly feel bad about yourself tomorrow if you lose one. Instead, abandon the notion of high and low self-esteem, because they're based on self-ratings. It works best not to rate yourself at all, either positively or negatively.

If you must rate something, rate and evaluate your *behavior,* not your *self.* When you stop esteeming or damning yourself as a whole, you can begin to fully accept yourself. You will begin to see yourself as a worthwhile human being who sometimes makes mistakes and acts badly. This is not to say that you shouldn't work to correct your mistakes or improve your behavior. Who do you think is more likely to pursue these goals? The self-accepting person is the one. The person who is convinced he's "rotten to the core" may not even try.

Try on the following belief statements. They are consistent with a new, healthier way of thinking. They reflect self-acceptance and positive self-esteem.

- Just because I succeeded or did not succeed today, that doesn't mean I will always do so in the future.
- It is wonderful to achieve and be approved of by others. But I don't need achievement or approval by anyone to feel good about myself.
- My performance at anything does not determine my worth as a human being.
- Everyone makes mistakes. I can accept myself while disliking and regretting my mistakes.
- Even though I may not like some of my traits and behaviors, I can still accept myself fully as a person.

Try adopting this realistic and self-accepting philosophy. Try practicing active listening and assertive responses. You may be able to improve your life and free your heart for its highest purpose: loving yourself and others.

Facts and Fallacies About Emotional Health

Stress is bad and unhealthy for me and I should really try to erase it from my life.

Some stress is necessary for good performance. It can provide a challenge, excitement, and meaning. The trick is to find just the right amount of stress for you. A life with too little stress would be boring and meaningless.

If I regularly practice relaxation techniques, I'll become so "mellow" and "laid back" that I'll get nothing accomplished.

"Laid back" does not necessarily mean "not ambitious." In fact, relaxation practice is energizing. In fact, you'll need to avoid practicing deep relaxation too close to bedtime.

I have many Coronary-Prone Behavior Pattern behaviors. I'm afraid that if I work to shift to more relaxed behaviors, I'll lose my drive and ambition.

Being relaxed does not mean that you are lazy or unmotivated. In fact, many relaxed and happy people are also ambitious and successful. They simply do not have the damaging stress that people with the CPBP tend to generate.

I suppose as a "Coronary-Prone Behavior Pattern" person I simply need to learn to "slow down and smell the roses" and not work so hard.

Working hard and moving quickly are not the most health-damaging aspects of CPBP behavior. Working to reduce your anger and hostility is the more important goal.

I'm a sales representative and have come to believe that the most aggressive person will usually win the prize. After all, we've all heard that "nice guys always finish last."

"Nice" does not necessarily mean "passive." Indeed, very passive people may frequently get the "short end of the stick." But assertive people can be "nice," yet have a much greater chance of success than very aggressive people do.

I think the best way to build up my self-esteem is to set goals and strive to accomplish them.

Although it is certainly great to accomplish goals, be careful about basing your worth as a person on your performance. Since everyone fails occasionally, you may feel rotten about yourself at these times. It is far better to strive for self-acceptance apart from achievement.

When I get very angry, the healthiest thing for me to do is blow up and get it out of my system as quickly as possible.

"Blowing up" (acting aggressively) may raise blood pressure, escalate the conflict, hurt relationships, and create feelings of guilt and anxiety in the aggressor. Instead, try to delay your response to a heated argument or conflict until you can calmly formulate an appropriate reply.

When I get very angry, it's best to try to appear very calm and not express it outwardly at all.

Some researchers believe that holding your anger in may be even more dangerous to your body than the more aggressive "anger-out" stance. An assertive, appropriately directed response is usually the best approach.

I have had numerous major life events and lots of daily hassles in the last few years. Does this mean that I can expect to develop a stress-related illness?

Not necessarily. Research suggests that your stress level is determined more by how you react and cope with stress than from the stress itself. If you do not regard the events of the past few years as particularly stressful to you, then they probably weren't.

The most important part of any good communication interaction is what I say and how I say it.

While a well-thought-out, assertive response is important, active listening is critical to good communication. If you don't understand the initial message, it won't matter how good your response is.

HIGHLIGHTS ——————————————

Easy Does It

As you saw in this chapter, there's no secret to a happy life. Simply accept yourself and others, live every day to the fullest, and work on reducing the negative stress in your life. You owe it to yourself—and to the people who love you.

PART THREE

HEART CONCERNS

Your Troubleshooting Guide

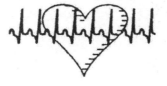

Chapter Nine

Troubleshooting

How to Spot Heart and Blood Vessel Problems

When you hear a knocking noise from under your car's hood, it's a good idea to check it out. The "Troubleshooting" section of your car owner's manual pinpoints symptoms and directs you to take specific actions to remedy the problem. Sometimes the problem is something you can fix; other times, you have to take the car to a mechanic.

This chapter is a troubleshooting guide for your heart and blood vessels. It is no substitute for regular medical checkups. It simply covers the symptoms of the most common heart and blood vessel problems and explains what to do about them.

Take a look at the "Troubleshooting Guide" below. The column on the left lists some symptoms of heart and blood vessel problems. Every symptom listed requires action. The column on the right directs you to the appropriate action. The text that follows the chart describes each action in detail.

TROUBLESHOOTING GUIDE

If You Feel	Take
Sudden pressure, fullness, squeezing, or pain in center of your chest lasting more than a few minutes, or that goes away and comes back	Action A
Pain that radiates from the center of your chest to your shoulders, neck, or arms	Action A
Chest discomfort with lightheadedness, fainting, sweating, nausea, or shortness of breath	Action A
Chest pain upon physical exertion or emotional excitement that usually goes away with rest and relaxation	Action B
Your heart beating suddenly very fast or in an irregular fashion	Action C
Sudden severe headache for no apparent cause	Action D
Sudden blurriness of vision or vision loss, especially in one eye	Action D
Sudden weakness or numbness of the face, arm, or leg or on one side of the body	Action D
Loss of speech or trouble speaking or understanding	Action D
Unexplained dizziness, unsteadiness, or sudden falls, especially along with any of the four previous sets of symptoms	Action D

Action A. Get help immediately! The symptoms listed are the early warning signs of a heart attack. If you experience one or more of these symptoms, do not delay. Call 911 or have someone drive you to the hospital. See "How to Get to an Emergency Room—Fast!" on page 304.

Action B. See your doctor at once, especially if you have never experienced these symptoms before. He will probably examine you for a condition called angina pectoris, or simply angina. Angina is chest pain resulting from a blockage in your coronary arteries. It must be treated as soon as possible. See "A Primer on Heart and Blood Vessel Problems," pages 293–299.

Action C. See your doctor immediately. If you feel your heart suddenly go from a normal beat to a very fast rate and it stays elevated for no apparent reason, tell your doctor immediately. If you feel your heart flutter or "flip-flop" numerous times in a short period of time, call your doctor without delay. This is especially important if you are experiencing any dizziness, nausea, or chest pain at the same time. You are probably experiencing an electrical problem called an arrhythmia. See "A Primer on Heart and Blood Vessel Problems," pages 293–299.

Action D. See your doctor immediately. The symptoms listed are the warning signs of stroke. Don't ignore these symptoms even if they seem to occur for only a minute or so. This may also indicate that you are experiencing a transient ischemic attack (TIA), a very strong predictor of stroke. For more information, see "A Primer on Heart and Blood Vessel Problems," pages 293–299.

A Primer on Heart and Blood Vessel Problems

Every heart owner should be familiar with the major problems that can affect the heart and blood vessels. Below, we've briefly outlined the most common conditions and diseases.

ANGINA PECTORIS (ANGINA). Angina is a type of pain that originates in the heart but is not a heart attack. It is a result of partial blockage in one or more of your coronary arteries, the vessels that feed blood to your heart.

Angina is a symptom of a condition called myocardial ischemia, or literally, "lack of blood flow (ischemia) to the heart (myocardium)." When there is not enough blood flowing into the coronary arteries, the amount of oxygen available to your working heart muscle is diminished. This is what causes the pain associated with angina.

To treat angina, it's necessary to reduce your heart's demand for oxygen. Drugs that slow your heart rate or reduce your blood pressure can decrease your heart's workload. Angina can also be treated by relaxing the coronary arteries and improving the flow of blood and oxygen to the heart. Sometimes coronary artery bypass surgery or other surgical techniques may be needed to improve the blood flow. Reducing or eliminating risk factors such as smoking, high blood pressure, high blood cholesterol, or obesity also can help to alleviate angina.

ARRHYTHMIA. Tiny electrical impulses normally regulate the beating of your heart. Arrhythmias occur when the transmission of these impulses is disrupted in some way.

There are many types of arrhythmias, ranging from those that are brief (and probably not noticeable) to others that last long enough to seriously affect your heart. When the latter occurs, the heart rate can slow to zero or race to high levels. In either case, the heart is not adequately circulating blood to the vital organs such as the brain and the heart itself.

These problems are made worse by underlying blood vessel problems such as atherosclerosis or high blood pressure. In this case, cardiac arrest or sudden cardiac death is possible.

Arrhythmias can also result from heart damage caused by:

- a congenital defect;
- scarring of the heart muscle caused by a previous heart attack;
- alcohol;
- cigarettes; or
- certain cardiac medications.

Arrhythmias may or may not require medical treatment. In general, before being treated, an arrhythmia must do one of the following. It must either cause severe symptoms or put you at risk of having more serious arrhythmias or future complications. Depending on the type of arrhythmia, treatments vary from drug therapy to surgery.

HEART ATTACK. A heart attack occurs when the blood supply to part of the heart muscle is severely reduced or stopped. This happens when one of the arteries that supplies blood to the heart muscle is blocked by an obstruction.

This obstruction is usually atherosclerosis, a build-up of fatty substances and cholesterol in the inner linings of the arteries. This build-up narrows the artery, slowing the flow of blood. Sometimes the obstruction is a blood clot that plugs up the narrowed artery. This is called a coronary thrombosis.

In either case, if the blood supply is cut off drastically or for a long time, muscle cells suffer irreversible injury and die. Disability or death can result, depending on how much of the heart muscle is damaged.

Richard loved Mexican food. He especially liked dishes with jalapeno peppers and hot chili sauce. The trouble was, spicy food didn't always agree with him. He often got a sharp pain in his chest shortly after eating a hot and spicy dinner. But he was fine after a couple of antacid tablets.

One evening after eating Mexican food, Richard again felt the familiar chest pain. He chewed two antacid tablets and waited for relief. But the pain got worse instead of better. After 20 minutes he started to sweat, and he felt nauseous.

"Oh, no," he thought, "I must have gotten food poisoning at that restaurant. I better lie down. Maybe it will go away."

His wife Karen arrived home an hour later and found Richard lying on the couch, barely able to speak. "I can't breathe," he said. "Feels like an elephant is standing on my chest."

Karen recognized the symptoms of a heart attack and immediately dialed 9-1-1. She explained Richard's condition to the operator. Waiting for the ambulance, Karen got Richard's medical records from the filing cabinet and called a neighbor to stay with the kids. Then she left a message for the family physician.

At the hospital, tests showed Richard was having a heart attack. Nearly two hours had passed since his symptoms began. The cardiologist told Richard he was lucky to be alive because he waited so long to get help. Miraculously, the damage to his heart was not severe. Richard underwent coronary artery bypass surgery a few days later to improve the blood flow to his heart. ●

HIGH BLOOD PRESSURE. If you have high blood pressure, your heart is working harder than normal to circulate your blood. This puts a strain on your heart and your arteries. High blood pressure can contribute to heart attacks, strokes, kidney failure, and atherosclerosis.

The biggest problem is that high blood pressure usually has no symptoms. In order to detect it, you must have your blood pressure checked regularly. There is no "ideal" blood pressure reading. But a reading below 140/90 mm Hg for adults is desirable. If your blood pressure reading remains at 140/90 mm Hg or higher for an extended period of time, you'll want to work with your doctor to lower it. This may require lifestyle changes. You may need to lose weight, cut down on salt, and limit alcohol intake. You may also need to get more regular exercise and take blood pressure medication.

Scientists don't know what causes high blood pressure in most cases. But we do know that keeping it under control is very important.

SILENT ISCHEMIA. Ischemia is a condition in which blood flow is restricted by a spasm or by clogged blood vessels. It can be painful, as in the case of angina. Or it may occur without any outward signs or warning. This is called *silent ischemia*.

People with silent ischemia may have a heart attack without any prior symptoms or warning. This problem can be detected by an exercise test or 24-hour heart monitoring.

SUDDEN CARDIAC DEATH. About half of all deaths from heart disease are sudden and unexpected. The victim may or may not have been previously diagnosed with heart disease. But the outcome is the same—the heart abruptly stops. This is called "cardiac arrest." Although the terms are often used interchangeably, a heart attack is rarely the cause of a cardiac arrest. More likely, in cardiac arrest, the cause is the heart beating rapidly and chaotically. This is called a life-threatening arrhythmia.

Regardless of the cause, cardiac arrest is reversible in most people if it's treated within a few minutes. Very often, this requires *defibrillation*. That uses an electrical impulse to shock the heart back into a normal rhythm. It can be done quite easily in a hospital or medical care setting. In fact, such facilities are well

298   YOUR HEART: *An Owner's Manual*

equipped for such emergencies. But outside of the hospital, the chance of surviving sudden cardiac death is remote without prompt cardiopulmonary resuscitation (CPR). (See "Your Number-One Lifesaving Technique: Cardiopulmonary Resuscitation," page 300.)

Fortunately, CPR can be provided by any person trained to do so. It doesn't require a medical professional. CPR keeps the blood circulating to the brain and to the heart muscle until the heart can be restarted by defibrillation. At that point, additional medical procedures may be necessary. These procedures may reduce damage to the heart or protect against fatal recurrences.

STROKE. A stroke occurs when a blood vessel bringing oxygen and nutrients to the brain bursts or is clogged by atherosclerosis or a blood clot. When this rupture or blockage happens, part of the brain doesn't get the flow of blood it needs. Then the oxygen-starved nerve cells begin to die within minutes.

When these nerve cells can't function, the part of your body controlled by these cells can't function either. With a stroke, you may lose your ability to walk, talk, see, remember, and even think. These devastating effects are often permanent because dead brain cells can't be replaced.

The greatest single cause of stroke is high blood pressure.

TRANSIENT ISCHEMIC ATTACKS (TIAS). About 10 percent of strokes are preceded by transient ischemic attacks. These are sometimes called "little strokes." About 36 percent of those who experience one or more TIAs will later have a stroke. Half of these people have a stroke within one year. Therefore, TIAs are very important warning signs of impending stroke.

A TIA occurs when a blood clot temporarily clogs

an artery, and part of the brain doesn't get the blood it needs. The symptoms of a TIA are similar to the warning signs of stroke. They usually last less than five minutes. When they go away, people tend to ignore them. This can be a deadly mistake.

If you experience these symptoms, get medical help immediately. Prompt medical or surgical attention could prevent a fatal or disabling stroke.

Heart disease runs in Clarence's family. Both of his grandfathers died of heart attacks in their 50s and his mother died of a stroke at 63.

At a recent medical check-up, Clarence was given a clean bill of health. But just as the doctor was about to leave the examination room, Clarence remembered to mention something. He told the doctor that several times in the last few months he had felt a little numbness in his right arm. It usually lasted less than a minute, then went away completely.

"I figure it's just muscle strain," said Clarence. "What can I do to keep it from happening again?"

The doctor was, of course, aware of Clarence's medical history. He suspected that the numbness was more than simply a muscle strain. When he questioned Clarence further, the doctor found that Clarence had severe headaches that would come and go.

"Clarence," he said, "I think that your symptoms may be the result of TIAs, or transient ischemic attacks. Some people call them mini-strokes." The doctor explained that TIAs are strong predictors of stroke. He said that if Clarence got treatment, he may be able to avoid a larger stroke. The doctor ordered several diagnostic tests. Then he put Clarence on a strict diet and medication. Two years later, Clarence has had no further problems. ●

Your Number-One Lifesaving Technique: Cardiopulmonary Resuscitation (CPR)

CPR is an easy-to-learn skill that can literally keep a person alive until additional medical help arrives.

CPR is a closed chest massage technique. It involves compressing the chest (and thereby the heart) in a rhythmic pattern. It also involves alternately forcing air into the victim's lungs by mouth-to-mouth breathing or *ventilation*. This keeps the heart and lungs working until the heart can be defibrillated.

Recently, with the advent of AIDS, some people have been concerned about CPR. They worry about becoming infected with HIV or other illnesses while doing CPR on a stranger. Some people even worry about being infected while learning how to perform CPR. But there has never been a documented case of HIV (or even hepatitis) transmitted during mouth-to-mouth resuscitation. In fact, scientists believe that AIDS is not transmitted through saliva.

Health professionals such as nurses, paramedics, and rehabilitation specialists give CPR regularly to strangers. They usually have mechanical ventilation devices, which tend to minimize possible infection. Remember that most episodes of sudden cardiac arrest occur in the victim's home. Therefore, as a CPR rescuer, you're likely to be with your own family members or friends. In this case, you would know if there was any risk of infection.

If you're trained in CPR, you could actually save the life of a family member or friend. If your family members are trained, they can help you, if you need it. For information on how you can learn CPR, call your local American Heart Association (see pages 386–388) or the American Red Cross.

With CPR, every second and every minute count. Any delay in giving CPR could result in the death or disablement of a person who might otherwise survive. Start CPR immediately and continue until emergency personnel arrive.

♥ Joan was a new dorm counselor at the local university. During Parent's Weekend she was assigned to register visitors as they arrived. She was busy filling out forms when someone in the registration line collapsed to the floor.

"Grandfather!" shrieked a male student, rushing to the man and kneeling beside him. "What's wrong?"

Joan rushed around the table and asked if she could help.

"He said he didn't feel well this morning," said the young man. "But he insisted on coming. He said he didn't want to miss our visit."

Joan could see that the man was pale and wasn't breathing. She asked someone to call an ambulance. She made sure that the man had not hurt his back or neck in the fall. Then she gently rolled him onto his back and immediately started CPR. She continued for nearly five minutes until the ambulance arrived.

A paramedic took over for her, while another examined the man. The paramedics asked people to step back. One then used the defibrillator to start the heart beating again. The other paramedic turned to Joan.

"Good work," he said. "We'll get him to the hospital now. Thanks to you, he'll probably recover without much damage."

On her way back to the dorm, exhausted and drained, Joan realized something. If this event had happened just two weeks earlier, she would have been as helpless as the other people in the room.

"How ironic," she thought. "When they told me I had to learn CPR to be a dorm counselor, I thought it was a stupid exercise. I thought it was useless—that I'd never need it. How wrong can a person be?" ●

When and How to Seek Emergency Help

If you've completed the "Heart Owner's Profile" on pages 5–11, you have an idea of your risk of heart attack. The truth is, a heart attack or stroke can happen to anyone.

If you or a loved one experiences any of the symptoms described in the "Troubleshooting Guide" on page 292, you know what to do. Remember, it's *critical* to get medical help fast. In fact, the faster the victim can get help, the greater the chance of reducing permanent damage and recovering quickly. This is true for both heart attack and stroke victims. To improve your odds, you must prepare in advance to handle a medical emergency.

Your risk of having a heart attack or stroke may be very high or relatively low. No matter what your risk is, you should still know how to make sure that you or a loved one gets prompt medical attention if needed. How ready are you to face a medical emergency? Find out by completing the following checklist.

YOUR MEDICAL EMERGENCY CHECKLIST

THE EARLY WARNING SIGNS OF HEART ATTACK OR STROKE

_____ You can easily identify all the early warning signs of a heart attack or stroke. (Quiz yourself by reviewing the symptoms to the left of "Action A" and "Action D" in the "Troubleshooting Guide" on page 292.)

YOUR EMERGENCY CARE RESOURCES

_____ What is the number for the emergency medical services in your community?

_____

Carry this number in your pocket, purse, or wallet. (Dialing "9-1-1" is all you need in many communities, but check to be sure. The time it takes to look up the phone number of the nearest ambulance service can cause a delay. That delay can be 30 seconds or up to two minutes. That could be the difference between life and death.)

_____ Which hospital emergency room is closest to your home? _

_____

Does this facility have an emergency cardiac care unit? _____ (Specialized care in such units has been shown to reduce in-hospital deaths by about 30 percent.)

Could you reach this facility faster if someone drove you instead of waiting for the paramedics? _____

_____ Which emergency room is closest to your work?

_____

Does this facility have an emergency cardiac care unit? _____ Could you get to this facility faster if someone drove you instead of waiting for the paramedics? _____

CARDIOPULMONARY RESUSCITATION

_____ You are currently trained in CPR.

_____ Members of your family who are trained in CPR: _____

_____

_____ Friends and co-workers who are trained in CPR: _____

_____

HOW TO GET TO AN EMERGENCY ROOM—FAST! When a medical emergency strikes, time is a life and death matter. Memorize the following checklist so that you can get help as quickly as possible.

EMERGENCY CHECKLIST

_____ If you think you may be suffering a heart attack or stroke, call emergency medical services first. Don't call your doctor for advice or guidance. Precious minutes can be wasted. The extra time such action takes may put you at increased risk for more extensive damage.

_____ If you are conscious and believe you can get to a nearby hospital more quickly than waiting for emergency medical service, *have someone drive you*. Never drive yourself! Try to remain calm. Anxiety and stress can make the problem worse.

_____ If you're with someone who is experiencing the symptoms of a heart attack, expect the person to deny that it's anything serious. Expect the person to make excuses ("it's only indigestion"). But don't take "no" for an answer. Insist on taking action. Get the person to a hospital emergency room immediately.

WHAT TO EXPECT IN THE EMERGENCY ROOM. If you're having a heart attack, the emergency room can seem confusing and scary. The good news is they know how to help you. Following is a step-by-step outline of what's likely to happen in the emergency room. There are also some suggestions that could help smooth your way.

- Go directly to the emergency room. If you are able, tell the attending medical staff:

    your symptoms,

    when the symptoms started, and

    how the symptoms have progressed since they started.

- The staff will hook you up to a continuous electrocardiogram (ECG or EKG) to monitor your heart. If the doctors think that you have suffered a heart attack, you may be moved to the coronary care unit (CCU). That is a special area of the hospital that specializes in treating heart attacks. If you suddenly go into cardiac arrest, the constant monitoring will enable the medical team to respond quickly to help you.
- Tubes will be inserted into your veins so that the medical team can easily give you medication.
- Depending on the initial test results, you may be given medication to dissolve a blood clot and restore blood flow. This procedure can reduce the extent to which the heart is permanently damaged. But the "clot busting" drugs are most effective very early in treatment (usually within one to three hours of when the heart attack begins). Therefore, any delay in recognizing early warning signs and seeking immediate medical attention can reduce their effectiveness.
- In the days or weeks that follow, your doctor may recommend one or more medical procedures. These may improve blood supply to the heart muscle. The next section, "If You Experience a Mechanical Breakdown," describes these and other procedures in more detail.
- If your symptoms indicate a possible stroke, physicians will perform a number of diagnostic tests. These tests determine the type of stroke and where in the brain it occurred. Treatment and rehabilitation will be individualized based on this information.

Are You a Survivor?

In many cases, the difference between surviving or succumbing to a heart attack or stroke is determined by a matter of seconds. Anything you can do to ensure prompt medical attention will help you to survive—and recover more fully. Start with the following advance plan.

- Know your own personal heart attack and stroke risk factors.
- Know the early warning signs of a heart attack or stroke.
- Be prepared to use the emergency rescue services efficiently and effectively.
- Know how to give CPR. Ask those around you to learn it, too.

Telephone Support

The telephone numbers below are those you can call for help with cardiovascular problems or emergencies. Please look up the numbers of your family physician or cardiologist and your local American Heart Association and fill them in, where indicated.

For emergency help in your community, call:

Police/emergency medical system .... 911.

For information, diagnosis, and treatment, call:

Your family physician or cardiologist ____-____.

For information on cardiovascular disease and how to help prevent it, call:

The American Heart Association .... 1-800-AHA-USA1.

Your local American Heart
Association .... ___-_____.

For information on where to learn CPR, call:

The American Heart
Association .... 1-800-AHA-USA1.

Your local American Heart
Association .... ___-_____.

The American Red Cross .... ___-_____.

HIGHLIGHTS ─────────────────────

Don't Borrow Trouble

On the other hand, don't overlook it. Simply review the symptoms listed in this troubleshooting guide from time to time. You may never experience them, but if you do, you'll know what's happening and how to get help. That knowledge could save your life.

PART FOUR

GENERAL REPAIRS

What to Do If You Have a Mechanical Breakdown

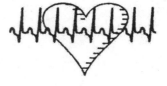

CHAPTER TEN

How to Find a Good Mechanic

 The Best Health Care

Even the best-running automobile will require regular tune-ups and minor repairs. If you wait until there's a breakdown to get this service, it can be inconvenient as well as expensive. When it's time for repairs, where do you go? Do you take your car to the dealer or a local garage? Do you try to fix the problem yourself or seek help from an experienced mechanic? And how do you find a really good mechanic?

Preventive maintenance and detecting problems early are even more important for your heart. First, you can start by taking care of yourself, so you can enjoy good health and a good quality of life. How? By practicing healthful habits such as not smoking, being physically active, eating nutritious foods, and managing those situations that are stressful for you. Another strategy that can save valuable time and money is to be prepared in case you do develop health problems. It may even help save your life.

This chapter will help you be a good medical care consumer. It describes the most common medical procedures used to diagnose and treat heart and blood vessel problems. It also suggests questions you should ask your doctor or health care provider.

How to Get the Most from the Health Care System

Every American is concerned about the availability and rising cost of health care. The following basic tips will help you get the best value for your health care dollar.

- Know what benefits are covered in your health care plan. Be sure you understand your managed care options, cost-sharing formulas and deductibles, and pre-authorization or pre-certification requirements.
- Keep good records of family medical information.
- Buy a simple health reference book and keep it handy. Look up information about symptoms and conditions before you call or visit a doctor or go to the emergency room. See Appendix B (on pages 380–385) for a list of resources.
- Take CPR and first aid classes.
- Use the emergency room only for emergencies. Explore other options for non-emergency needs, such as outpatient services or after-hours clinics.
- Always check your billing statements to be sure you are not charged for services you did not receive.

 ## How to Choose a Doctor

It's a good idea to have a primary care doctor to handle most of your basic health care needs. A primary care doctor is usually a family practitioner, a general internist, or often a gynecologist. He or she can help you find a specialist if you need one. In fact, many health care plans require that your primary care doctor refer you to a specialist before the plan will cover the specialist's bill.

A few of the specialists who may be involved with problems associated with your heart include the following.

- Anesthesiologist—Decides the type of anesthesia to be used during surgery, administers it, and monitors its effects after surgery.
- Cardiologist—Diagnoses and treats problems of the heart and blood vessels.
- Exercise Physiologist—Evaluates fitness levels and plans and supervises exercise programs.
- Internist—Specializes in diagnosing and treating nonsurgical adult medical problems.
- Registered Dietitian—Plans diets and educates patients about healthful dietary habits.
- Cardiovascular Surgeon—A general surgeon who specializes in the diagnosis and surgical treatment of abnormalities of the heart and blood vessels.
- Respiratory Therapist—Develops breathing exercises to help patients avoid respiratory infections following surgery in the chest.

How you choose a doctor may depend on your health care plan. Your plan may allow you to choose any doctor you wish. Your plan may also assign you to a doctor or provide you with a list of doctors for you to choose from. But no matter how you select your doctor, he or she should be licensed and in good standing. If you don't know any doctors, ask friends and family members for their recommendations. Contact the nearest county medical association for a list or brochure containing the names of board-certified doctors in your area.

Before you make an appointment for your first visit, call the doctor's office and ask the receptionist the following questions.

- Is the doctor accepting new patients?
- For routine visits, how far in advance must you make an appointment?
- What hospital does the doctor use?
- Does the office accept your health insurance plan?
- What is the doctor's fee for an office visit?
- How long has the doctor been in practice?

If you are satisfied with what you learn, schedule an appointment with the doctor for an interview or a routine exam. Be prepared for your first visit.

- If you're changing doctors, have your medical records sent ahead in advance.
- Make a list of questions that are important to you. Don't be afraid to ask the doctor to explain further if you don't understand technical terms.
- Bring along a list of medications you are taking

After your visit with the new doctor, evaluate your experience.

- Was the facility clean and pleasant?
- Were the staff friendly and professional?
- Were patient education materials or programs available?
- Did the doctor seem to be a caring person?
- Did the doctor explain things in a way that was easy to understand?
- Did the doctor encourage you to ask questions?

If your experience was not what you wanted it to be, consider your alternatives. You may want to talk to the doctor about your concerns. If you are still not satisfied, you may want to find out if your health care plan allows you to choose another doctor. If it does, you may consider switching doctors. If your plan does not allow this, share your concerns with your plan administrator.

Doctors are not your only source of health information. In fact, people get health information from a variety of sources. This includes many outside the medical care system, such as television, newspaper, magazines, friends, and family members. Unfortunately, not all of the health information available from these sources is technically sound or accurate. Also, you may be justifiably concerned about the reliability of new medical discoveries and treatments.

So how can you be a responsible health care consumer? A good way to start is by applying the following questions and criteria to any health information that you read or hear. They should help you sort fact from fiction.

- Is the recommendation or treatment based on scientific studies?
- How effective is the recommended treatment compared to other treatments, or to doing nothing at all?
- Have the studies been subjected to scientific review and published in respected medical journals?
- Are citations provided that include the name, location, and credentials of the investigators?
- How well controlled were the studies?
- Were the treatment groups compared with groups not receiving the treatment?
- Have the studies been repeated with the same results obtained in other situations?
- How many people were studied or received the proposed treatment or therapy?

- What percentage of those who tried the therapy have actually been helped?
- Was there some other possible explanation for the results that were obtained?
- How safe is the treatment or remedy?
- Do the benefits associated with the treatment outweigh the potential risks?
- Are words such as "miracle," "breakthrough," and "cure" used in the advertisement? If so, it is probably too good to be true.
- Is the product sold only through the mail or door-to-door? These methods are usually used by people or groups who have to "get out of town fast" when consumers discover that their product is fraudulent.

 ## What You Should Know About Drugs and Medication

Medications are a serious matter. You should understand them fully before you agree to take them. Many doctors make it a policy to explain the benefits and possible side effects of drug therapy before writing a prescription. If your doctor does this, you needn't read any further.

But if your doctor is quick to prescribe drugs, but does not offer a rationale, you may want to ask some questions. The ones below will help safeguard your body as well as afford you peace of mind. Ask your doctor these eight questions before you accept any written prescription.

1. What's the generic and the trade name of this drug?
2. How strong is it?
3. Why do you think I should take this drug?

4. Are you sure it will interact positively with the other medications I'm taking? (Be prepared to list everything you're taking, from other prescription drugs to over-the-counter medications, even vitamins.)
5. How do you recommend I take this drug? (For example, with meals or on an empty stomach? With water or juice?)
6. What side effects should I be watching out for? Should I report them to you right away or wait until our next visit?
7. Are there any activities—such as driving a car or operating machinery—that I should not do while taking this drug?
8. How long do I have to take this drug?

MEDICATION LABELING AND STORAGE TIPS. Before leaving a pharmacy, make sure that a prescription's label contains the following items.

- The pharmacy's name, address, and phone number
- Your name, spelled correctly
- The prescription number
- The name of the medication, and whether it's a trade name or generic
- Directions about how much of the drug to take, and when
- Expiration date, if applicable
- Your prescribing doctor's name
- The current date
- Any special storage instructions

Proper storage is important. Medications that aren't handled correctly can lose their effectiveness. In addition to heeding the drug manufacturer's or your pharmacist's instructions, keep in mind the following storage tips.

- Bathrooms are often humid, so don't store medications there. Instead, find a storage place in a room where the humidity is low and the temperature is fairly constant.
- Store all medications in their original containers with the labels securely affixed.
- Never combine different tablets or capsules in the same container, even to make it easier to carry them in your pocket or purse, or when you're traveling. If you become incapacitated and someone else has to give you your medication, the right labeling information is critical.
- If necessary, ask your pharmacist for smaller labeled containers that are easier to carry around.
- Don't put medicines in your car's glove compartment. And don't leave them on a windowsill or anywhere they are exposed to direct sunlight. Excessive heat or cold can sometimes affect the ingredients.
- All medicines should be kept well out of children's reach.

MEDICATIONS LIST. Make a chart like the one below to keep track of your medications. Take this list with you to doctor appointments, trips to the pharmacy, and when you buy over-the-counter medications.

MEDICATIONS LIST

Name of Medication: Start Date:

Doctor's Name: End Date:

Prescribed for:

Dosage: _____ taken _____ times per day for _____ days.

Special Instructions or Precautions:

OTHER SAFETY TIPS ABOUT MEDICATIONS.

- Take the full amount of your prescription. Even if you start to feel better, don't stop unless you are specifically told otherwise by your doctor. Find out what to do if you should miss a dose of your medicine.
- Take the medicine only as directed. For example, coated tablets must not be chewed, crushed, or dissolved in water. They must be swallowed whole. The purpose of the coating is to allow the medication to be released at a specific point in the digestive tract. Capsules should also be swallowed whole.
- Ask about how alcohol may interact with medications you are taking.
- Never take another person's prescription.
- Flush any unused or expired prescription medicines down the toilet. Rinse out and throw away old medicine bottles. Never use them to store other medicines.
- Watch for expiration dates on over-the-counter drugs.

HIGHLIGHTS

What's Up, Doc?

Now that you know the ins and outs of health care plans, choosing a doctor, and dealing with medications, let's take a look at various diagnostic procedures. These procedures help your doctor determine your condition and formulate the most effective treatment.

CHAPTER ELEVEN

How to Diagnose Heart and Blood Vessel Problems

If necessary, you can make major repairs to your car's engine to correct mechanical problems and extend your car's life. In the same way, doctors can make major repairs to your heart and blood vessels that will restore health and vigor if you're suffering from coronary heart disease. In the most extreme case, your "engine" could be replaced by having a heart transplant.

Yet, the medical treatment procedures described on the following pages are serious measures. They should not be considered lightly or viewed as a "fix" or "cure" but as an opportunity to change what caused the heart problem in the first place.

 ## Understanding Diagnostic Procedures

Medical technology has made spectacular advances during the past thirty years. Today, medical specialists have a variety of tools and tests they can use to pinpoint heart problems with astounding accuracy. These tests range from a routine physical examination to sophisticated nuclear medical techniques. All are intended to determine the amount of damage to the heart muscle or the risk of future heart damage.

As a result of these tests, a doctor may decide to continue a patient's current medication or medical treatment. Or the doctor may recommend corrective surgery or angioplasty (balloon dilation). Or you may be able to solve the problem with lifestyle change and rehabilitation. This chapter reviews some of the more common ways to diagnose and treat cardiovascular disease.

ELECTROCARDIOGRAM OR ECG. The purpose of the ECG is to measure the electrical activity of your heart. This test can be performed while you're resting or while you're exercising. At rest, the heart's oxygen requirements aren't that great. So the heart may be able to compensate for any slowdown due to clogged coronary arteries. This is why resting ECG tests may give a person a clean bill of health when, in fact, he or she may have severe coronary artery disease.

The obvious way around this problem is to get your heart to require more oxygen by making it work harder during the ECG monitoring. An exercise stress test (Figure 13) can reveal a great deal to the doctor. It can be useful in diagnosing heart problems and in prescribing safe and effective exercise programs.

Before an exercise stress test, you'll be asked to follow the following procedures.

- Get no strenuous activity on the day of the test.
- Eat no food for two or three hours before the test.

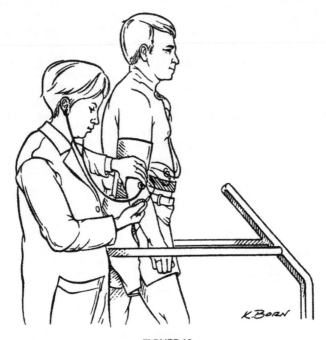

FIGURE 13
Exercise Stress Test

- Dress for exercise. Wear comfortable walking shoes and loose-fitting clothes.
- Review all current medications with your doctor.
- Learn and understand the benefits and risks of the exercise test and perhaps sign an informed-consent form. (This is the time to ask any questions about the test.)

In the exercise lab, a nurse or technician will apply disks, called electrodes, to various points on the front of your upper body, and sometimes on the back. First, however, your skin must be cleaned with alcohol and lightly scrubbed with fine sandpaper where the electrodes will make contact. Men often have their chest hair shaved where the electrodes will be placed. This improves the quality of the ECG recordings. Generally it takes ten or more electrodes, referred to as leads, to allow the heart's electrical activity to be monitored from various directions.

Once the electrodes are in place, the technician connects them to a series of wires that are hooked up to an electrocardiograph machine. Before the test begins, the nurse or technician will take your blood pressure reading. Then they will take your resting ECG with you in two positions (lying down and standing). This will show them if any irregularities occur with a change in positions. The doctor may ask you to hyperventilate by breathing deeply and rapidly for at least 20 seconds. These procedures help eliminate the chances of a false-positive test—a test that appears to be abnormal, but is not.

DO YOU NEED A STRESS TEST?

The American Heart Association recommends an exercise stress test under the following conditions:

- If you are a sedentary person over age 40 and you are going to participate in a vigorous exercise program.

- If you are under age 40 and you have risk factors for or a strong family history of coronary heart disease.

- At any age, if you have cardiovascular disease or its symptoms, lung disease, or a metabolic disease such as diabetes or hyperthyroidism, see your doctor before starting any type of exercise program. He or she will decide if you need a stress test.

Exercise stress tests can be performed on treadmills or stationary cycles. In the United States, treadmills are more commonly used.

Several common exercise test protocols are used. The protocol tells the doctor how to conduct the test—how fast the treadmill should run, for what length of time, and the angle of the treadmill (grade). The test is divided into several stages, each progressively more challenging. Each stage requires a change in speed and/or grade. The protocol also indicates exactly how much energy you should be expending during each stage of the test.

You are encouraged to communicate with the testing staff at all times during the test. The doctor will stop the test when you reach a preset maximal heart rate, when abnormal symptoms are noted, or if you complain of pain or serious fatigue.

At the end of the test, hold on to the front bar of the treadmill as it slows down and levels off in grade. After a brief cool-down period, you'll lie down again, this time for six to ten minutes. During this time the staff continues to monitor blood pressure and ECG at regular intervals during the recovery period.

How safe is an exercise stress test? It is quite safe, even for people with cardiovascular disease. A physician who is experienced in performing and interpreting the ECG should always be immediately available during an exercise stress test.

NUCLEAR MEDICINE TECHNIQUES. The following diagnostic techniques offer cardiologists a way to look deep inside your heart to determine its condition and to recommend the proper treatment.

Radionuclide Ventriculography. If the cardiologist suspects that the left ventricle of your heart is not working correctly, he or she may order a radionuclide ventriculography.

In this specialized nuclear cardiology test, a tiny amount of radioactive isotope is injected into your bloodstream. These radioactive isotopes are safe because they decay so quickly that they remain in the body only long enough for the test to be completed.

When the radioactive material passes through your heart, the doctor can accurately measure the percentage of blood the left ventricle ejects when it contracts. This percentage is called the ejection fraction. The normal resting ejection fraction for the left ventricle is about 60. Any reading less than 45 percent indicates severe left ventricular dysfunction. This shows a high risk for future heart problems.

Thallium Scan. Another nuclear medicine technique that can improve upon the accuracy of an exercise test is a thallium scan. It is commonly used after a heart attack to find out how much of the heart was damaged.

Here's how it works. Toward the end of an exercise test, you are injected with thallium-201, a radioactive isotope, through an intravenous line. Immediately after exercise, doctors can see the parts of your heart where the blood supply is inadequate because the thallium will not reach those areas. He or she can also see those areas where your heart attack occurred.

Three or four hours after the exercise test, he or she remeasures the thallium. This distinguishes those areas that were temporarily blocked from areas of the heart muscle that were permanently damaged during the heart attack. Thallium will still be present only in the damaged part of the heart muscle.

Echocardiography. This is an ultrasound procedure that bounces sound waves off the surface of your heart. The results are converted into "pictures" that the cardiologist can read. This procedure can also be used to estimate the left ventricular ejection fraction, but is less accurate than a radionuclide ventriculography.

Holter Monitoring. This diagnostic procedure is used when the doctor suspects left ventricular dysfunction. This monitoring technique helps determine if you are having frequent irregular heartbeats or "PVCs" (premature ventricular contractions).

With Holter monitoring, you wear a small tape recorder for at least 24 hours, usually on a belt around the waist. This monitor records the heart's electrical signals. They can be played back later using special equipment that helps single out those fleeting heart rhythm disturbances that aren't captured during an ordinary ECG.

Angiogram or Angiography. Angiography is designed to find out if you need specialized heart surgery. A coronary angiogram pinpoints the actual sites of narrowing in your coronary arteries and gives the surgeon a road map to follow if surgery is necessary.

Angiography can be performed on an inpatient or an outpatient basis. The doctor usually orders a few preliminary tests, including a chest x-ray, ECG, and blood workup before the angiogram.

About an hour before the exam, you'll get a sedative to help you relax. The angiogram will be performed in a special room called a cardiac catheterization laboratory ("cath lab") by a cardiologist. You simply lie on a table under an X-ray camera, and you're hooked up to an ECG monitor. The area where the catheter will be inserted is shaved, cleaned, and anesthetized with a local anesthetic.

You'll remain fully conscious while the cardiologist

inserts a thin plastic tube into an artery in your groin or arm. The doctor gradually moves the catheter up the artery to the arteries in the heart. Then the doctor injects a dye into the coronary arteries while an X-ray machine shoots a rapid series of pictures. Next, the catheter is placed inside the left ventricle and dye is injected there as well. This procedure is called left ventriculography and is routinely performed during coronary angiography.

Usually, you won't feel the catheter moving through your arteries. But you may feel a sensation of warmth or tingling when the dye is released. It's important that you are conscious during this procedure because the doctor will ask you to take a few deep breaths and hold them or to cough.

Throughout the angiography, either you or the X-ray camera will be moved into various positions so that the doctor can view your heart and arteries from different angles. As the physician is viewing what's happening on the TV monitor, the X-rays are being recorded on a videocassette. You can watch the monitor, too, if you like.

The entire procedure generally takes about an hour, but this can vary depending on your condition, what the doctor is checking for, and many other factors. When it's over, medical personnel will remove the catheter and apply pressure over the area of insertion to prevent bleeding. Sometimes it's necessary to take a stitch or two.

Within twenty-four hours after the angiogram, almost all of the dye is excreted from your body through your kidneys. If you're stable after the test, you'll be discharged and can return to full activities the next day.

Coronary angiography is an extremely safe procedure. When the procedure is performed correctly, the death rate is less than 0.2 percent and the risk of heart attack, stroke, or severe bleeding is less than 0.5 percent.

HIGHLIGHTS

What's Next?

After your doctor has diagnosed your heart or blood vessel problem, he or she will recommend a treatment plan. It may be that medication alone will take care of the problem. Other times, your condition will require a medical procedure or surgery. In the next chapter, we'll look at the most common heart and blood vessel treatments.

CHAPTER TWELVE

Medical and Surgical Repair Techniques for Heart Disease

 What You Can Expect to Gain

Your cardiologist will use the results of your angiogram and left ventriculography, as well as other pertinent information, to diagnose your condition. Then he or she decides whether you are a suitable candidate for an angioplasty or coronary artery bypass surgery. Your cardiologist considers the following factors in making a final decision:

- Symptoms
- Age
- Exercise ECG results
- Left ventricular functions
- Number of narrowed coronary arteries
- Sites and severity of plaque buildup in the coronary arteries

The basic goal of angioplasty or bypass surgery is the same. That is to reestablish an adequate blood supply to areas of the heart muscle that have become deprived over the years because of blockages in the coronary arteries. An angioplasty achieves the goal by widening the coronary arteries at the sites where they've become narrowed by plaque. Bypass surgery gets the same results by detouring the blood around the narrowed parts of the coronary arteries.

Angioplasty

Nearly 400,000 angioplasties are performed each year in the United States, and the success rate is more than 90 percent. In a small percentage of patients, the dilated coronary artery will become blocked again within about six months and the procedure may need to be repeated.

Angioplasty has the following advantages over bypass surgery.

- It requires a shorter stay in the hospital.
- It's a less radical procedure.
- There are fewer complications.
- It costs less than bypass surgery.

At the same time, not all coronary artery disease patients are candidates for angioplasty. Patients with blockage in a single artery usually respond well to angioplasty, except when the blockage occurs in the left main coronary artery. Blockage in this area is most risky, and bypass is the favored treatment for this condition.

The procedure for angioplasty is similar to the angiogram procedure. Angioplasty is performed in the cath lab and you are awake and prepared in much the same way. The cardiologist inserts a catheter through your arm or groin and guides it into the coronary artery under constant X-ray monitoring.

Here's where the procedures differ. A second catheter is passed on the inside of the first catheter into the coronary artery. This second catheter has at its end a small, tough deflated balloon. The cardiologist injects dye into the artery to help guide the balloon-tipped catheter into the narrowed areas. The doctor inflates the balloon within each of the blocked areas to flatten out the plaque and open up the coronary artery (see Figure 14). Immediately after the balloon is de-

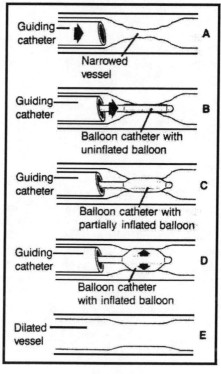

FIGURE 14
Angioplasty

flated, an angiogram is performed to determine if the angioplasty has done the necessary job.

After the angioplasty procedure, you'll be observed closely for several hours. The place where the catheter was inserted may be bruised and a little sore. With no complications, you'll be free to leave the hospital in a few days and can resume normal activity almost immediately.

How safe is angioplasty? Complications are rare. In less than five percent of the people having angioplasty, emergency coronary bypass surgery is required. For this reason, even though the chance for emergency surgery is remote, angioplasty must be performed only in a setting where an emergency heart surgery team is on standby.

Martha was fifty-one years old when she decided to join a fitness club. The club required that she have an exercise stress test before being admitted as a member.

Although she thought it was unnecessary, she had the ECG stress test. She was stunned when the technician said that he couldn't release her for the exercise program because there was an abnormality in the test. The technician referred Martha to a doctor, who explained that an exercise stress test didn't, by itself, confirm the presence of heart disease. A few days later, Martha had an angiogram. Blockage was discovered in one coronary artery. The doctor said that Martha was a good candidate for angioplasty.

Martha had the angioplasty procedure and has fully recovered. She joined the fitness club and exercises regularly. She has also made other positive changes in her lifestyle to prevent heart problems in the future. ●

Coronary Artery Bypass Surgery

Considerable controversy surrounds the long-term benefits of bypass surgery. But most doctors agree that bypass surgery does prolong life and improve the quality of life. The challenge is to determine whether a given patient should have bypass surgery or if angioplasty would do just as well.

Because bypass surgery is more radical and expensive than angioplasty, your doctor will carefully weigh the benefits and risks before recommending this procedure. Bypass surgery is often advised for people with blockage in the left main coronary artery or in people with left ventricular dysfunction.

The goal of bypass surgery is to detour blood around a blocked coronary artery. Increased blood flow should eliminate the chest pain (angina pectoris) that occurs with exercise. It will also greatly increase the ability to exercise. Other benefits include reducing fatigue, cutting the need for medication, and restoring a sense of well-being.

OPEN-HEART SURGERY. Coronary artery bypass surgery is an open-heart operation. It involves removing part of an artery or vein from another part of the body and sewing (or grafting) it onto the heart's arteries. In this way, a blocked area is bypassed. The arteries or veins used in this operation are not essential ones Removing them doesn't significantly affect the blood flow where they're taken.

Typically, the surgeon uses one of two blood vessels as grafts. One is the saphenous vein (a superficial vein that runs down the inside of the leg). The other is an internal mammary/thoracic artery (vessels down the right and left side of the chest alongside the breast bone). There are merits to using each, and most cardiac surgeons use a combination of both types of vessels.

During surgery these arteries or veins are connected directly to the coronary arteries on the surface of the heart. The connections are made in front of and behind the blockages. This way, blood flows through them, bypassing the narrowed or closed points.

WHAT TO EXPECT AT THE HOSPITAL. As you would expect, preparing for bypass surgery is more extensive than preparing for angioplasty. As a coronary artery bypass patient, you'll be under a general anesthetic during the operation, which takes about four to six hours depending on the complexity of your condition. Coronary artery bypass operations are performed using a heart-lung machine. This machine makes it possible to stop the beating motion of your heart, until the grafts can be precisely connected to the tiny coronary arteries.

After the operation is completed, you'll remain in the cardiac intensive care unit for twelve to twenty-four hours. You'll be connected to a respirator and numerous other tubes and wires during this period. You'll barely be aware of it, however, because you'll be on pain medications that will keep you asleep most of the time.

After a day or two you'll be taken to a room on the cardiac floor, where your condition will be closely and continuously monitored. Of course, you'll have some chest discomfort and some leg pain if the saphenous veins were used. A respiratory therapist will work with you on deep breathing exercises to help clear your lungs of fluid and prevent pneumonia. Most people are amazed at how fast they get up and move around. After about a week or two, you'll be discharged from the hospital and continue your rehabilitation at home.

WHAT TO EXPECT AT HOME. The wounds from bypass surgery usually heal within about three to six weeks. It takes about eight weeks for the sternum (which was cut to open the chest cavity) to heal completely. You shouldn't pull, push, or lift any object weighing more than ten pounds during this period. Wearing elastic stockings may help reduce pain in your legs and feet and prevent swelling. Aspirin therapy or anti-platelet treatment may be prescribed to prevent occlusion of the bypass vessels.

During the rehabilitation period, you'll usually have "good days" and "bad days," with overall progress and a gain in strength. Being active is a good way to regain your strength. Walking is especially beneficial after bypass surgery. Gradually increase the time and distance you exercise every day without overdoing it.

Exercise also helps relieve depression, which is common when a person first returns home. The emotional letdown after any operation may cause such feelings. You may think you're not progressing fast enough. Time may seem to stand still. It's a good idea to talk with family members and friends regularly because this helps fight depression. It's important that your family members be careful not to add to the depression. These feelings usually subside as you resume your normal activities.

Jerry had coronary artery bypass surgery and progressed well. Four weeks after the surgery he entered the second phase of his cardiac rehabilitation program. Jerry was eager to resume his normal activities, including driving the car, climbing stairs, and working in the yard. His doctor said he was progressing well and would be able to resume vigorous activities soon.

Jerry and his wife Norma were a little embarrassed to ask about resuming sexual activity, but they finally asked the doctor about it. The doctor talked with Jerry and Norma about their sexual preferences and explored ways to help them ease the transition to intercourse. They were surprised to learn that more than 75 percent of heart patients don't change their former patterns of foreplay or sexual position after a heart attack or heart surgery.

The doctor said that sexual activity after heart surgery was quite safe if you have sex with your usual partner in comfortable surroundings. He explained that the energy expended in sex is about the same as walking up two flights of stairs. Jerry and Norma agreed to talk about their feelings and needs openly and honestly.

At his next doctor's visit, Jerry was happy to report that he and Norma had reaffirmed their relationship and that it was even fuller and richer than before the surgery. ●

Heart Valve Surgery

You have four heart valves. Their job is to ensure that blood flows forward as your heart contracts and relaxes. A human heart beats more than 100,000 times each day. So its valves must flex, stretch, and hold back pressure hundreds of millions of times in an average lifetime.

Heart valves may not always work as well as they should. Several things can cause problems and require repairs.

- A heart valve may not be normal at birth and require immediate repair.
- A minor defect that exists at birth may cause problems later in life.

- Diseases such as rheumatic fever or bacterial infections may cause scarring or damage to the valve.
- The aging process may weaken or harden the valve.

Any problem with a heart valve greatly increases your heart's work. That may cause the heart to enlarge to make up for its extra workload. When the heart can no longer do that, heart failure soon follows. Over time the heart muscle is permanently damaged.

Some people with diseased heart valves can lead normal lives as long as they get careful medical supervision. Others, with more severe heart valve damage, need surgery to repair or replace the valve.

Operations to repair valves are the most natural way to treat valve failure because your own valve tissues are used. But sometimes the valves are so seriously deformed, degenerated, or destroyed that this is not possible. The old, damaged valve must be removed and replaced with a new valve.

TYPES OF HEART VALVES. Several types of replacement valve mechanisms are used. Biological tissue valves use animal valves or the aortic valve from a human donor. Tissue valves have the great advantage of being very similar to the natural heart valve it replaces. These valves are well tolerated in the body without special medications. The disadvantage is that they're usually less durable than mechanical valves.

Mechanical valves are artificial devices made of hard and durable metals. Although their durability is a distinct advantage, these valves aren't natural to the body so they may cause blood clots to form. To keep this from happening, people with mechanical valves must take medication every day for the rest of their lives.

WHAT TO EXPECT DURING VALVE SURGERY. If you're having heart valve surgery, you will experience many of the same procedures and feelings as other heart surgery patients. Heart valve operations usually take three to five hours, depending upon the complexity of the case. Generally, you'll be released one to two weeks after surgery.

Respiratory therapy is an important part of your initial recovery process. You'll do deep breathing exercises and vigorous coughing to help clear out the fluids that often collect in the lungs during and after heart surgery. Starting while you're in the hospital, you'll participate in a cardiac rehabilitation program that includes a gradual exercise program. Most people can walk two to three miles a day within a few weeks after their operation.

SPECIAL CONSIDERATIONS. If you received a mechanical valve, you'll take medication to prevent blood clots from forming on these artificial devices. These medications are often called "blood-thinners," but they're more accurately described as "anticoagulants." They don't really thin the blood; they just slightly prolong its clotting time. If you're taking anticoagulants, follow your doctor's instructions very carefully and take medicine exactly as prescribed. These medications must be taken daily and at the same time each day. They also must be carefully monitored at regular intervals by taking a blood test called a prothrombin time ("protime").

If you have a heart valve problem, you must inform your dentist and other doctors about their condition so that antibiotics can be prescribed before and after procedures that are likely to cause bleeding. Otherwise, bacteria could be released into the bloodstream during these procedures and cause an infection in the heart called bacterial endocarditis. Doctors and dentists also need to know if you are taking anticoagulant medications because they may need to make adjustments to prevent excessive bleeding. If this is the case, be sure to carry an ID card in your wallet to alert health professionals to these conditions.

HEART VALVES BRING NEW LIFE. Too often, people with heart valve disease are disabled. Heart valve surgery holds the promise of a better quality of life. Most patients find that after an operation they can do many things that were impossible before. As with other surgeries, successful recovery depends on following medical advice, which includes exercise and other forms of healthy living.

How risky is heart valve surgery? Repairing heart valves or replacing them with prosthetic valves are reliable operations. Problems are rare, but they sometimes do happen. That's why it's important for patients and their families to plan ahead to take immediate action in case of a medical emergency that relates to the heart valve.

What You Should Know About Pacemakers

An artificial pacemaker is a twentieth century wonder. It's medical science's solution to the electrical problem of a slow heartbeat.

Your heart has a natural pacemaker, which produces electrical impulses that cause it to contract and pump blood. Impulses normally travel from the pacemaker cells down certain electrical paths in the muscle walls. As long as these impulses occur at regular intervals, your heart pumps at a rhythmic pace.

But problems can arise that change your heart's rhythm. Your heartbeat may be slow and often irregular. Or it may sometimes be normal and sometimes too fast or too slow. In either case blood isn't being pumped around your body efficiently. An artificial pacemaker may be recommended to make your heart beat more regularly so that enough oxygen and nourishment can get to your body's cells.

HOW A PACEMAKER WORKS. There are two parts of an artificial pacemaker system. The pacemaker generator is a small battery-powered unit that produces the electrical impulses that start the heartbeat. The generator is implanted under your skin through a small incision. It's connected to the heart through tiny wires that are implanted at the same time. The impulses flow through these wires (leads) to the heart and are timed to slow at regular intervals just as impulses from the heart's natural pacemaker normally do.

Most pacemakers work only when they're needed. They're called "demand pacemakers." Demand pacemakers have a sensing device that shuts off the pacemaker if the heart beats faster than a certain rate. When the heart is beating slower than the pacemaker rate, the sensing device turns the pacemaker on again. In this way, a demand pacemaker works something like a thermostat. The difference is that instead of working according to temperature, it works according to the heart rate.

CARING FOR YOUR PACEMAKER. As with any electronic device, the pacemaker requires care. From time to time, the batteries must be replaced through a minor surgical procedure. The doctor will regularly monitor the pacemaker to detect if the batteries are running down. If you have a pacemaker, you'll be taught to take your pulse to check that your heart is pumping correctly. Also, you'll need to tell other doctors, dentists, and health professionals that you have a pacemaker.

Modern pacemakers have built-in features to protect them from most types of interference produced by other electrical devices, such as microwave ovens, televisions, vacuum cleaners, hair dryers, etc. Most office and light shop equipment such as computers, typewriters, copy machines, and woodworking and metalworking tools also pose no risk to pacemakers. The metal detection devices in airports may detect a pacemaker, but won't damage it. However, high-current industrial equipment and powerful magnets may affect how a pacemaker works.

How risky is having a pacemaker? Having a pacemaker implanted is a relatively simple procedure, not nearly as invasive as the coronary bypass or heart valve surgery described above. Installing a pacemaker takes about an hour and the procedure usually requires a short stay in the hospital.

Today many thousands of people have pacemakers and lead full, productive lives. Self-monitoring, taking medications as prescribed, and seeing your doctor regularly are the keys to living with a pacemaker.

What You Should Know About Heart Transplants

When a heart is so damaged that it can't be repaired, current treatments may not be able to relieve the symptoms and prolong life. When all hope for improvement is lost, a heart transplant should be considered.

In a heart transplant, the diseased heart is removed and replaced with a healthy human heart. In special cases, the diseased heart may not be removed. Instead, a surgeon may put a healthy heart next to the diseased one (a "piggy-back" heart transplant) to act as a booster pump.

The first human heart transplant was performed in December 1967 by Dr. Christiaan Barnard in Capetown, South Africa. In the early years, heart transplants usually weren't successful because the patient's body often "rejected" the new heart. Now, because we have a better understanding of how the immune system works, survival rates after a heart transplant have gradually improved.

Today, almost 2,000 Americans have heart transplants every year in more than 150 heart transplant centers. The current results are encouraging.

- Four out of five patients are expected to survive one year.
- Seven of ten will still be alive five years after their operation.
- Almost half of those who receive a transplant today will survive more than ten years.
- The longest survivors are alive more than twenty years after their transplant.

Heart transplants are reserved for people who have a high risk of dying from heart disease within one to two years. Transplants can be done on newborns as well as people in their 70s. Most transplant patients have one of these problems:

- Irreversible damage to the heart from hardening of the arteries (coronary artery disease) and multiple heart attacks
- Damage to the heart muscle cells, which impairs the heart's ability to contract normally (cardiomyopathy or heart muscle disease)
- Abnormalities in the heart valves that cause injury to the heart muscle
- Abnormalities of the heart muscle or other structures that exist at birth (congenital heart disease)

When deciding whether a person would be a good candidate for a heart transplant, doctors consider the following factors.

- The amount of damage or disease in other organs (brain, lungs, liver, kidneys) that can't be repaired
- Evidence of other medical problems, such as active infection, diabetes, or blood clots in the lungs
- Ability to deal with the emotional strain of a transplant and its aftermath
- Ability to cope with potentially serious side effects from medications
- Need for lifelong treatment and medical care
- History of active drug or alcohol abuse
- Network of supportive family or friends
- Mental illness

It's estimated that at least 15,000 people each year in the United States could benefit from a heart transplant. Unfortunately, only about 2,000 hearts a year are available for transplantation.

Donor hearts are given to patients based on the following:

- Donor's blood type and body weight
- Potential recipient's blood type, body weight, and severity of illness
- Geographic location (seriously ill recipients at a nearby transplant center are given priority)

A suitable heart donor is a young to middle-aged person who's been declared brain dead based on standard criteria and whose heart still works well. Most donors give multiple organs. All donors are screened to make sure the Hepatitis B and C and human immunodeficiency (HIV, or AIDS-producing) viruses aren't present. Any evidence of these infections means a person does not qualify as an organ donor.

When a transplant team from the recipient hospital is notified of a suitable heart, they travel quickly to the donor hospital. There they remove the heart and put it in a special cold solution to keep it alive (even though it's not beating). A heart can be disconnected from a person's circulation for about four hours without losing its ability to work properly. Thus, time is critical. When the heart is removed, the team returns to their hospital and performs the operation.

The most common early complications after a heart transplant are organ rejection and infection. Doctors can detect early rejection long before the patient feels anything or before there's any active sign of the heart not working normally. Although anti-rejection drugs must be continued for life, the dose may be reduced six to eight months after the transplant. That will help reduce or eliminate the side effects of the drugs.

The steps taken to protect against rejection may increase the risk of infection. The same white blood cells that attack the transplanted heart are responsible for removing foreign particles (such as bacteria) from the circulation.

After the first year, the major threat to survival comes from blockages that develop in the arteries of the transplanted heart. If the blockages progress, abnormalities in how the heart muscle works or irregularities in heart rhythm may develop. In such cases, a second transplant operation may be considered.

FUTURE DIRECTIONS OF CARDIAC TRANSPLANTATION. Heart transplantation has improved dramatically in the past twenty years. New options are constantly being studied. Researchers are working on the following.

- New anti-rejection drugs for preventing rejection with fewer side effects
- Techniques to diagnose rejection without a heart biopsy
- Treatment and prevention of blockage in the vessels of the new heart
- Other heart replacement options—artificial heart pumps or mechanical support systems or xenograft (transplant organs of other species)
- Greater access to donor organs
- Early identification of heart disease and treatment to stop the disease before a transplant is needed

THE PROCESS OF HEART DONATION. The process of donating and receiving a heart is a simple, but exacting process. It works like this:

- The potential donor signs an organ donor card.
- Following brain death, the donor's relatives are contacted.
- Consent is given by the next of kin.
- Determination is made of the acceptability of the heart, lungs, liver, kidneys, cornea, bone, and skin for possible transplantation.
- Recipients are identified and prioritized via a local transplant program or the UNOS (United Network for Organ Sharing) computer.
- The recipient is notified and admitted to the hospital.
- Surgical teams from the transplant center arrive at the donor hospital at a predetermined time.
- The surgical removal of the donor organs is begun.
- The recipient is taken to the operating room, where removal of the diseased heart is coordinated with the arrival of the donor organ.

HIGHLIGHTS ————————————————

Now That Your Heart Problem Is Repaired

Repairing your heart is only the beginning. As the next chapter will show, wise heart patients start cardiac rehabilitation immediately and continue those good habits for the rest of their lives.

CHAPTER THIRTEEN

Heart Attack and Stroke Rehabilitation

 Recovering from a Heart Attack or Heart Surgery

Cardiac rehabilitation is designed to restore a person who has had a heart attack, angioplasty, or heart surgery to optimal physiological and psychological health. A good, comprehensive recovery program includes exercise training, psychological counseling, vocational counseling, and behavioral change to modify cardiovascular disease risk factors.

Two phases of cardiac rehabilitation are:

- Phase 1—Inpatient Program
- Phase 2—Outpatient Program

Additional programs are available for people who cannot take advantage of a Phase 2 outpatient program. These people may, on advice of their physicians, take part in a long-term community-based program or an unsupervised maintenance program.

Based on a patient's history and any complications

347

that may have arisen, doctors can predict the likelihood of future cardiac events. The doctor uses this information and his or her best judgment to classify each patient as low-, moderate- or high-risk. The patient's risk level guides the cardiac rehabilitation team in developing his or her individualized program, including the timelines for each of the phases. Here are the characteristics of each phase and the activities included in each.

PHASE I

- Usually begins within 24 to 48 hours after the attack or procedure.
- Aims to prevent the adverse effects of bed rest.
- Provides medical surveillance for patients while they begin to undertake normal daily physical activities.
- Prepares patients for the more vigorous phase that follows.

While a good in-patient program is individualized to each patient's needs, the following activities are typically included.

- Range of motion activities while still in bed
- Sitting, standing, and walking exercises
- Climbing stairs
- Light handheld weights (one to three pounds per hand)

The overall goal of Phase 1 is to keep the exercise intensity low, gradually increasing the duration of the exercise sessions. All Phase 1 exercise sessions are always supervised by a nurse, physical therapist, exercise physiologist, or some other qualified health professional.

PHASE 2

- Usually begins immediately after hospital discharge and lasts for four to twelve weeks.
- Aims to continue to reverse any reduction in fitness caused by hospitalization and bed rest.
- Attempts to get the patient adjusted and committed to a structured, medically directed exercise program.

The following activities are usually included.

- Patients exercise three to five times a week in a hospital or some other local health facility.
- Sessions usually last 30 to 60 minutes and include stretching exercises, calisthenics, light weight training, walking, and stationary cycling.
- Heart rate remains relatively low throughout, not exceeding 85% of the rate that was attained during the most recent submaximal exercise test.

Ideally, there should be at least one health care staff member present for every five patients exercising during a Phase 2 program. Low-risk patients in rural or remote areas where there is no organized exercise program can implement their own program at home. But moderate- or high-risk patients must be supervised. In progressing to long-term community-based programs, angioplasty patients generally do best, followed by bypass surgery patients. Heart attack sufferers must be most cautious of all.

LONG-TERM COMMUNITY-BASED PROGRAMS. Your doctor will advise you whether you can participate in long-term community-based programs after you have completed your outpatient program. The program:

- Begins six to twelve weeks after hospitalization (always a minimum of six weeks for bypass or heart attack patients).

- Aims to maintain the fitness gains achieved during Phase 2 and make more progress toward normalcy.

These programs are conducted in local community facilities, including YMCAs, Jewish community centers, fitness centers, private rehabilitation centers, or university medical schools. They are not necessarily held in medical facilities. Doctor referrals are required to join these programs, and patients must present the results of an exercise stress test before beginning. The patient-to-staff ratio can be higher than in Phase 2, but should never exceed a ratio of ten to one. Staff members conducting these programs should be trained to read participants' ECGs and to handle emergencies.

Exercise activities in these groups are similar to those in Phase 2, including the following.

- Patients exercise three to five times a week.
- Sessions usually last 30 to 60 minutes and include stretching exercises, calisthenics, light weight training, walking, stationary cycling, swimming, and perhaps noncompetitive activities such as volleyball. Patients at low risk are given more freedom to regulate their own exercise.
- Heart rates do not exceed 85% of the rate that was attained during the most recent maximal exercise test (should be higher since the Phase 2 test was a submaximal test).

UNSUPERVISED MAINTENANCE PROGRAMS. An unsupervised maintenance program is a medically directed program. People who participate in this kind of program are often people who have dropped out of a long-term community-based program. They drop out usually because of individual preference, economic concern, geographic isolation, or reasons related to convenience rather than to health. The program:

- Begins after at least three months in a medically supervised rehabilitation program.
- Requires no on-site medical supervision.
- Follows exercise guidelines approved by the patient's doctor.

An unsupervised maintenance program's exercise prescription usually includes the following.

- Patients exercise three to five times a week.
- Sessions usually last 30 to 60 minutes and include stretching exercises, calisthenics, light weight training, walking, jogging, stationary cycling, swimming, low-impact aerobics, and perhaps noncompetitive team sports.
- Because the exercise is unsupervised, the heart rate limit may be set slightly lower than it was during the long-term community-based program.

WHAT ABOUT DIET? As part of your cardiac rehabilitation program, the doctor, dietitian, or nursing staff will help you learn how to modify your eating style. Heart disease risk factors such as high blood cholesterol and high blood pressure, and contributing factors such as obesity and diabetes, can be affected by changes in diet. As a heart patient, you'll usually be advised to do the following.

- Reduce the fat in your diet, especially saturated fat and cholesterol
- Reduce salt intake
- Keep calorie intake at an appropriate level to achieve and maintain a healthful body weight

Moderation and common sense usually are the best guides in both eating and drinking. For more information about a heart-healthy diet, see Chapter Four, "Healthy Nutrition—The Right Fuel for Your Tank," on pages 57–128.

WHAT ABOUT BLOOD CHOLESTEROL? Nutrition experts generally agree that keeping your blood cholesterol at a desirable level reduces the risk of heart complications if you have coronary artery disease. During your recovery and rehabilitation period, the doctor will check your blood cholesterol from time to time. If it's too high and if proper diet and exercise can't bring it within a normal range, then you may need medication.

WHAT ABOUT SMOKING? Smoking is a major risk factor for additional heart disease after surgery. If you're a heart patient who smokes, you are strongly encouraged to quit. A smoking cessation program is an important part of cardiac rehabilitation for smokers.

OTHER LIFESTYLE HABITS. You may want to consider changing other aspects of your lifestyle habits. Only you can decide what's right for you. For example, doctors often recommend that you take steps to reduce stress and tension in your life by doing the following.

- Avoid self-imposed and external deadlines and a preoccupation with time
- Learn to cope with situations that regularly cause angry or hostile feelings
- Increase your leisure time activities
- Improve communication with family and friends

After a relatively minor angioplasty procedure, Jenny was feeling great. Her improvement was dramatic—she could walk up stairs without feeling winded and out of breath. She thought her heart problems were behind her.

For the first couple of years after the angioplasty, Jenny was serious about her rehabilitation. But slowly her lifestyle habits began to slip. Before she knew it, she had returned to her old way of cooking and eating. She had quit exercising and gained 20 pounds.

Fortunately, she went to her doctor for a routine checkup. Her doctor was alarmed at how much her blood cholesterol level had increased. He explained that reverting to her old habits could cause her arteries to become clogged all over again. Jenny is now back on her rehabilitation program, exercising regularly, and eating the low-fat way. She now understands that heart-healthy habits must be a lifetime—not a short-time—commitment. ●

BEYOND REHABILITATION. It is important that you use your cardiac rehabilitation program as an opportunity to learn and practice new skills of healthy living. Sticking with your exercise program once it's started is critical. Regrettably, many cardiac patients drop out of their exercise programs within a year. The critical dropout period is the first three to six months.

The following tips have helped many patients stay active beyond rehabilitation.

- Know the benefits of exercising and the risks of not being active.
- Start slowly and progress gradually.
- Find ways to make physical activity convenient.
- Choose a form of exercise that you enjoy.
- Join an exercise group or find a partner.
- Find a role model and, later, serve as a role model for others.
- Plan ahead to anticipate and compensate for those situations in which it will be difficult to exercise.
- Obtain support from family members and friends.
- Look for ways to be active through your lifestyle pursuits—gardening, household chores, playing with children, etc.

Dave and Earl are sheet-metal workers who put in long hours. Both men have a great deal of job-related stress. At times, they've both been known to express anger and hostility.

Unfortunately, they both ended up in the cardiac care unit of the local hospital following heart attacks. After an appropriate stay in the hospital, both were released to continue their recovery at home. They even attended the same cardiac rehabilitation program.

Earl consistently attended the program activities and progressed well. Friends and family members noticed that he had adopted a new attitude. He seemed less angry. He had rechanneled his energy toward his rehabilitation program and regaining productivity.

Dave, on the other hand, attended a few cardiac rehab classes, then dropped out because he got too busy. Before long he was back to leading a tense and stressful life, feeling angry and hostile much of the time.

Earl was surprised to hear that Dave was back in the hospital again and this time his heart attack was extremely serious. If only Dave had stuck with the rehabilitation program. Earl felt good that he had used rehabilitation as an opportunity to change the things about his lifestyle that got him into trouble in the first place. ●

Recovering from a Stroke

Rehabilitation after a stroke is extremely individualized because each stroke patient is different. No single rehabilitation program is right for everyone who has experienced a stroke.

EXERCISE. Exercises are important. They prevent your muscles from getting too tight, and they help you regain full use of your body. Here are some basic tips about post-stroke exercises:

- Consult your doctor before starting any exercise program after stroke.
- Don't exercise too hard in the beginning.
- Try to build up strength and endurance gradually.
- Your exercise program should start with:
   —improving flexibility and muscle tone, including stretching and relaxation programs such as yoga
   —strengthening exercises recommended by your physical therapist or doctor
   —pleasure walking
   —other activities such as gardening, golf, housework, or yardwork

Some stroke survivors can pursue more vigorous activities. Check with your doctor. The most important thing is to enjoy the exercise program you choose. Use common sense not to push yourself too hard.

MEDICATION. If you're a stroke survivor, you may get pains in your shoulder and hand on your weaker side. Usually the physical effects of stroke can be reduced by doing exercises, taking medications, or using special equipment. Here's some advice about medication:

- Understand the directions and purpose for the medicine.
- Establish a system for taking medicine correctly and monitoring the process.
- Ask about alternatives if your medications are difficult to swallow.

SPECIAL EQUIPMENT. Braces, splints, or special equipment may be prescribed for different reasons. A leg brace or arm sling may give you support. A wrist splint may prevent deformity. A spoon with a special handle may replace some lost ability. As a stroke survivor, you can benefit significantly from these adaptations. Remember to:

- Use the devices until the doctor or therapist says it's okay to stop.
- Have your equipment checked regularly to make sure it works properly.

OTHER CONSIDERATIONS. You may have other problems and frustrations during your recovery process. Comprehensive medical care and your own ability to be patient with yourself will help you adapt to changes in your body and find new ways to do daily tasks. So will support from your family members. Stroke clubs and support groups for stroke survivors exist in many areas. You'll benefit greatly from opportunities to socialize, share feelings, and find out how others are coping with similar problems.

The following tips can also help you through the recovery process.

- Find new interests or hobbies and enjoy leisure time.
- Check out "talking" books at the library.
- Learn about access for the handicapped in public places. Guides are usually published by the Chamber of Commerce in major cities.
- Inquire about benefits and services from Medicaid or Medicare from the local Department of Social Services.
- Contact the State Office of Vocational Rehabilitation if there is interest in vocational retraining.
- Contact the doctor or other health team member if there are symptoms of stroke-related problems.

● After her stroke, Elaine had some serious adjust-
♥ ments to make. So many of the simple tasks of
living seemed impossible. She really tried to be
patient, but she couldn't help getting frustrated with
herself and her family.

Over time, this frustration led to depression. Her
family became concerned enough to speak to her
doctor. The doctor suggested antidepressant medications and careful monitoring. Soon the family noticed
that Elaine's mood seemed to improve. She began to
try to do more for herself and started to make progress.

The family was greatly relieved. Now they felt they
were all back on track. But they knew they had a lot to
learn about stroke and depression. Elaine's illness,
it was clear, had affected them, too. With Elaine's
agreement, the whole family joined a stroke support
group. It felt good to know others who had similar
needs and to feel they weren't alone. ●

HIGHLIGHTS

Learning to Live the Good Life

*Heart and stroke patients who succeed at rehabilita-
tion don't stop there. They adopt a healthy lifestyle
and stick with it—for life.*

*Take a look at the Appendix. You'll find dozens
of ways to get involved in life again. Join the AHA's
Mended Hearts, Inc., or The Stroke Connection support group. Or volunteer for the American Heart
Association and other heart-related community organizations.*

It will do your heart good.

APPENDIX A

Maintenance Schedules and Service Logs

The owner's manual for your car has places in it for you to record information about any service or scheduled maintenance that you have done to your car. Use the forms in this appendix to help you keep track of the maintenance information that is important to the health of your engine. Blood pressure, blood cholesterol, and weight management logs are included. Also included are forms to help you change habits to reduce your risk for heart disease and stroke. Guidelines for using each form are described below. Make photocopies of the forms so you can track your habits for several days or weeks.

 Dietary Tracking Log

There are two parts to this tracking form: the Food Record and the Daily Variety and Balance Checklist. Follow the instructions below for each part.

PART I: FOOD RECORD. Use this portion of the form to record everything you eat and drink and the circum-

359

stances under which it was eaten. Also record the nutrient information for the amount of the food or beverage that you actually consumed. The following suggestions may help you improve the accuracy of your record-keeping.

- Write down each food immediately after you eat it. Carry the form with you at all times so you don't have to rely on memory.
- Use one line for each food. If a certain dish has many components (such as a ham and cheese sandwich), put each component (bread, cheese, ham, mayonnaise) on a separate line.
- Describe the foods fully. For example, for baked chicken, was it baked with the skin on and, if so, did you eat the skin?
- Be very specific about portion size. If necessary, use measuring tools (cups, spoons, weight scales) to determine exact amounts.
- Use the "Nutrition Facts" label from the packaged foods you eat to calculate nutrient content. Also, special food reference books are available at most bookstores.

PART II. DAILY VARIETY AND BALANCE CHECKLIST. Use this part of the form to keep track of the number of servings per food group you eat for the day. The number of servings that you should eat in each food group is represented by a circle shape (one circle equals one serving). For each serving you eat, put a check mark inside the shape in the corresponding food group. Try to eat the minimum number from each food group every day.

You can choose to eat more servings, especially from the Breads and Vegetables and Fruits groups, if desired. Keep track of "extra" servings by filling in the "□."

Serving Sizes

Breads, Cereals, Pasta, and Starchy Vegetables

1 slice of bread
½ bagel
½ hamburger, hot dog
  bun
¼–½ cup starchy
  vegetables

¼ cup nugget or bud-type
  cereal
½ cup hot cereal
1 cup flaked cereal

Dietary Tracking Log

Date: _____

PART I. FOOD RECORD

Time/ Place/ Person(s)	Food Description	Amount Eaten	Calories	Fat (g)	Choles- terol (mg)	Other*
Daily Totals						

*Can be used to track saturated fat, sodium, or other nutrients of specific interest to you. You can also use this space to record emotions, thoughts, or events that precede or follow your eating events.

PART II. VARIETY AND BALANCE CHECKLIST

Breads, Cereals, Starchy
Vegetables
(Six or more servings a day)
○○○○○○
□□□□□

Lean Meats, Poultry, Fish
(No more than two servings a
day)
○○   □

Vegetables and Fruits
(At least five servings a day)
○○○○○○
□□□□□   □□□□□

Fats and Oils
(Eat sparingly)
□□□□

Low-fat Milk and Dairy
Products
(Two or more servings a day)
○○
□□

Desserts, Sweets, Snacks
(Eat sparingly)
□□□□

Vegetables·

¾ cup vegetable juice
1 cup raw leafy greens

½ cup chopped or cooked

Fruits

1 medium piece
½ cup fruit juice

½ cup sliced or canned
¼ cup dried (raisins,
   apricots)

Low-Fat Milk and Dairy Products

1 cup milk
1 cup yogurt

1 oz. hard cheese
½ cup cottage cheese

Lean Meat, Poultry, Fish, Dry Beans

3 oz. cooked (4 oz. raw)
1 cup cooked dry beans, peas, lentils

Physical Activity Tracking Log

Use this form to keep track of all the physical activities you do throughout the day. Record "programmed exercise" such as working out at a gym, riding your bike at the park, walking in the neighborhood before work, etc. Also include moderate-level "lifestyle" physical activities such as taking the stairs at work, vacuuming, working in the yard, etc.

The bottom part of the form will help you keep track of how balanced your physical activity is. It is important to include all types of activities (aerobic, strength, and flexibility) throughout the week.

- Aerobic
  - Walking
  - Cycling
  - Jogging
  - Swimming
  - Vacuuming
  - Stair climbing
  - Raking
- Strength and Toning
  - Calisthenics (push-ups, stomach crunches, pull-ups)
  - Weight training (weight machines, hand weights)
- Flexibility
  - Stretching exercises

Physical Activity Tracking Log

Date: _____

Time	Place/Person	Physical Activity	Duration	Other*

*Use this column to record physical activity intensity level, emotions, thoughts, or events that precede or follow your physical activity.

BALANCED FITNESS LOG
Put a check (✓) beside each part of a balanced fitness program that you completed today.

____ Aerobic (Walking, Cycling, Jogging, Swimming, Stair climbing, Raking, Vacuuming, etc.)
____ Strength and Toning (Calisthenics and Weight Training)
____ Flexibility (Stretching Exercises)

Smoking Habits Log

If you smoke, this log will help you track your use of tobacco products. Fold and attach with a rubber band a copy of this form to your cigarette pack. Every time you smoke a cigarette, fill in one line on the form. If you get the urge to smoke, but don't actually light up, record that, too, on the form.

Review several days of records to look for patterns in your smoking habits. For example, look at the following elements.

- Time of day;
- Duration between cigarettes;
- Places where you smoke the most;
- People or activities associated with your smoking habits; and
- Your feelings before and after you smoke a cigarette.

Use the information you get from tracking to help you pinpoint ways to make quitting smoking more successful.

Smoking Habits Log

Date/Time	Place/Person	Activity	Feeling(s) Before	Feeling(s) After

Date/Time	Place/Person	Activity	Feeling(s) Before	Feeling(s) After

Blood Cholesterol Log

This graph will help you keep track of your blood cholesterol level checkups and the results. It will enable you to easily see how your cholesterol levels change over time.

Each time you have your cholesterol checked:

- Write in the date of the blood test on the horizontal axis. Then plot the new level on the graph. Connect the new level to the most recent level with a straight line.
- Record total, HDL, and LDL cholesterol. Simply use different color pens or different icons to distinguish between the different values.

Remember, if you are 20 years old or older, you should have your total and HDL cholesterol levels tested at least once every five years. Your physician may recommend more frequent testing, depending on your cholesterol level or other heart disease risk factors.

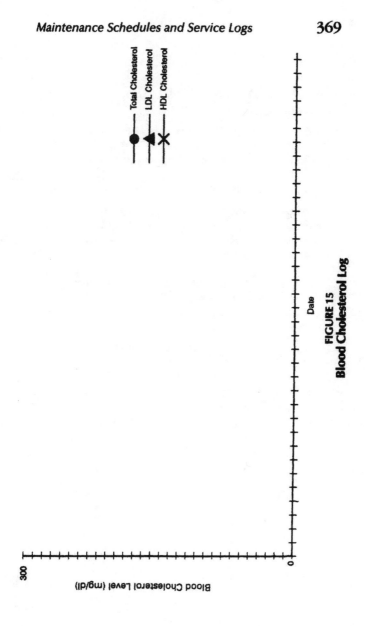

**FIGURE 15
Blood Cholesterol Log**

Blood Pressure Log

Like the blood cholesterol log, recording your blood pressure on the graph provided can, at-a-glance, give you a summary of your blood pressure history. You complete it much in the same way as the blood cholesterol graph.

Each time you have your blood pressure checked:

- Write in the date of blood pressure test on the horizontal axis. Then plot the new reading on the graph. Connect the new reading to the most recent reading with a straight line.
- Record both your systolic (the higher number) and diastolic (the lower number) blood pressure levels. Simply use different color pens or different icons to distinguish between the different types.

If your blood pressure is normal, you should have it checked at least every two years. If it is slightly above normal, you should have it checked once a year. Your doctor will tell you if you need to get it checked more frequently.

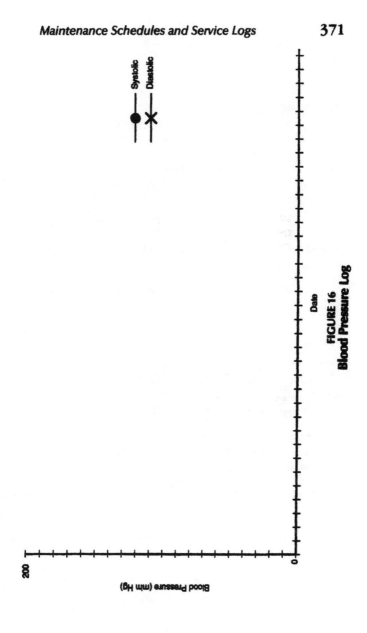

FIGURE 16
Blood Pressure Log

Body Weight Log

Have you ever been surprised at your annual checkup when your doctor tells you that you have gained two pounds? Then the next year you come back and you have gained two more pounds—without even knowing it. It's easy to let slow weight gain creep up on you.

This graph will help you track your weight. It can be an especially motivating tool if you are trying to lose weight. Keep the following suggestions in mind.

- Weigh no more frequently than once a week. It is best if you weigh yourself only once a month or less.
- Weigh yourself at the same time of day.
- Wear the same amount of clothes when you weigh (i.e., don't weigh naked one time and with all your clothes on the next).

Keep track of your weight by using this log.

- For your first entry, write down the date on the spot of the horizontal axis farthest to the left. Then, on the vertical axis, put your weight at the level that says, "Starting Weight."
- In descending one- or two-pound increments, write in other weights on the vertical axis.
- On subsequent entries, write in the date on the horizontal line, plot the new weight on the graph, and connect the new weight and the previous weight with a straight line.

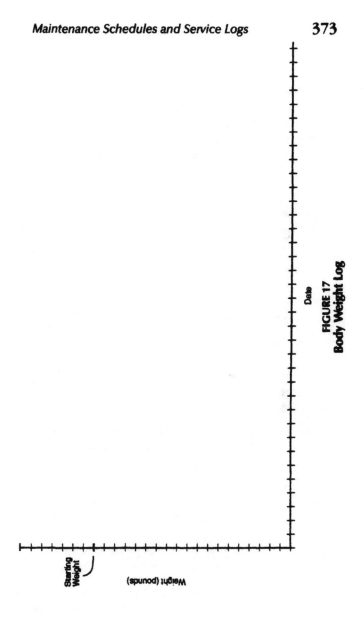

FIGURE 17
Body Weight Log

Heart Disease and Stroke Risk Reduction Contract

Use this simple form to guide you through the goal-setting process. If necessary, continue your planning on separate pages. Having someone witness your contract is not necessary. But some people find it helpful to be accountable to another person.

Heart Disease and Stroke Risk Reduction Contract

I, _____, pledge that I will

_____

_____

on or before _____.

This goal is: Mine ____ Realistic ____ Measurable ____

My plans and mini-goals for attaining this goal are:

I will ask _____ to help me by

_____.

I will reward his/her efforts by _____.

I will review (and modify, if necessary) my goals and plans on the following dates: _____

When I attain my goal, I will reward myself by _____

_____.

| _____ | | _____ | |
| Signature | Date | Witness signature (optional) | Date |

The American Heart Association recommends cardiovascular health education and intervention for parents and health care providers according to the following schedule.

Age	Pediatrician's Responsibility	Parent's Responsibility
0–2 years	• Obtain family history for early heart disease and stroke; if positive refer parent for further evaluation on risk factors. • Start growth chart. • Inform parent about heart-healthy diet for parents and older children in the family.	• If smoker, quit. • Change from breast-feeding or formula to whole milk at approximately one year. • Have nutritious snacks on hand.
2–6 years	• Update family history and growth chart (educate parent about concept of height and weight ratio). • Start blood pressure chart at approximately 3 years of age; review concept of lower salt intake with parent if necessary. • Determine blood cholesterol levels if child has positive family history or if one parent has a total cholesterol level >240 mg/dl. If the child's level is abnormal, counsel parent on dietary changes.	• Start low-fat (less than 30 percent of daily calories from fat), low-cholesterol diet. • Change to low-fat and nonfat dairy products. • Play actively with child.

(continued)

Age	Pediatrician's Responsibility	Parent's Responsibility
6–10 years	• Update family history, blood pressure and growth charts. • Do a complete cardiovascular health profile with child: family medical history, smoking history, blood pressure percentile, weight for height, total cholesterol, and level of activity and fitness.	• Continue heart-healthy diet. • Begin active anti-smoking education. • Encourage life sport activities that child and family can enjoy. • Limit television watching if child is very sedentary.
>10 years	• Update family history, blood pressure, and growth charts annually. • Consider measuring total cholesterol, HDL cholesterol, LDL cholesterol, and triglycerides in all patients.	• Review heart-healthy diet, risks of smoking, benefits of physical activity whenever possible. • Model heart-healthy behaviors.

 ## CHART FOR SCORING THE ONE-MILE FITNESS TEST

MEN—ASSUMES A BODY WEIGHT OF 175 POUNDS

Age	Heart Rate	Low Fitness	Moderate Fitness	High Fitness
20–29	110	>19:36	17:06–19:36	<17:06
	120	>19:10	16:36–19:10	<16:36
	130	>18:35	16:06–18:35	<16:06
	140	>18:06	15:36–18:06	<15:36
	150	>17:36	15:10–17:36	<15:10
	160	>17:09	14:42–17:09	<14:42
	170	>16:39	14:12–16:39	<14:12

Age	Heart Rate	Low Fitness	Moderate Fitness	High Fitness
30–39	110	>18:21	15:54–18:21	<15:54
	120	>17:52	15:24–17:52	<15:24
	130	>17:22	14:54–17:22	<14:54
	140	>16:54	14:30–16:54	<14:30
	150	>16:26	14:00–16:26	<14:00
	160	>15:58	13:30–15:58	<13:30
	170	>15:28	13:01–15:28	<13:01
40–49	110	>18:05	15:38–18:05	<15:38
	120	>17:36	15:09–17:36	<15:09
	130	>17:07	14:41–17:07	<14:41
	140	>16:38	14:12–16:38	<14:12
	150	>16:09	13:42–16:09	<13:42
	160	>15:42	13:15–15:42	<13:15
	170	>15:12	12:45–15:12	<12:45
50–59	110	>17:49	15:22–17:49	<15:22
	120	>17:20	14:53–17:20	<14:53
	130	>16:51	14:24–16:51	<14:24
	140	>16:22	13:51–16:22	<13:51
	150	>15:53	13:26–15:53	<13:26
	160	>15:26	12:59–15:26	<12:59
	170	>14:56	12:30–14:56	<12:30
60 +	110	>17:55	15:33–17:55	<15:33
	120	>17:24	15:04–17:24	<15:04
	130	>16:57	14:35–16:57	<14:36
	140	>16:28	14:07–16:28	<14:07
	150	>15:59	13:39–15:59	<13:39
	160	>15:30	13:10–15:30	<13:10
	170	>15:04	12:42–15:04	<12:42

For every 10 lbs. over 175 lbs., men must walk 15 seconds faster to qualify for a fitness category.

For every 10 lbs. under 175 lbs., men can walk 15 seconds slower and still qualify for a fitness category.

WOMEN—ASSUMES A BODY
WEIGHT OF 125 POUNDS

Age	Heart Rate	Low Fitness	Moderate Fitness	High Fitness
20–29	110	>20:57	19:08–20:57	<19:08
	120	>20:27	18:38–20:27	<18:38
	130	>20:00	18:12–20:00	<18:12
	140	>19:30	17:42–19:30	<17:42
	150	>19:00	17:12–19:00	<17:12
	160	>18:30	16:42–18:30	<16:42
	170	>18:00	16:12–18:00	<16:12
30–39	110	>19:46	17:52–19:46	<17:52
	120	>19:18	17:24–19:18	<17:24
	130	>18:48	16:54–18:48	<16:54
	140	>18:18	16:24–18:18	<16:24
	150	>17:48	15:54–17:48	<15:54
	160	>17:18	15:24:17:18	<15:24
	170	>16:54	14:55–16:54	<14:55
40–49	110	>19:15	17:20–19:15	<17:20
	120	>18:45	16:50–18:45	<16:50
	130	>18:18	16:24–18:18	<16:24
	140	>17:48	15:54–17:48	<15:54
	150	>17:18	15:24:17:18	<15:24
	160	>16:48	14:54–16:48	<14:54
	170	>16:18	14:25–16:18	<14:25
50–59	110	>18:40	17:40–18:40	<17:04
	120	>18:12	16:36–18:12	<16:36
	130	>17:42	16:06–17:42	<16:06
	140	>17:18	15:36–17:18	<15:36
	150	>16:48	15:06–16:48	<15:06
	160	>16:18	14:36–16:18	<14:36
	170	>15:48	14:06–15:48	<14:06
60+	110	>18:00	16:36–18:00	<16:36
	120	>17:30	16:06–17:30	<16:06
	130	>17:01	15:37–17:01	<15:37
	140	>16:31	15:09–16:31	<15:09
	150	>16:02	14:39–16:02	<14:39
	160	>15:32	14:12–15:32	<14:12
	170	>15:04	13:42–15:04	<13:42

For every 10 lbs. over 125 lbs., women must walk 15 seconds faster to qualify for a fitness category.

For every 10 lbs. under 125 lbs., women can walk 15 second slower and still qualify for a fitness category.

Credits: Adapted with permission from Living With Exercise by Steven N. Blair, P.E.D., Director of Epidemiology at the Cooper Institute for Aerobics Research in Dallas. (Dallas: American Health Publishing Company, 1991, 1-800-736-7323). All rights reserved. The One-Mile Fitness Test is based on maximal oxygen uptake estimates from studies done by Dr. James M. Rippe and colleagues. JAMA 1988; volume 259:2720-2724.

APPENDIX B

For Further Information

Note: Listed below are organizations, companies, books, periodicals, and videocassettes that may provide information of interest to you. Inclusion in this list does not constitute an endorsement, implied or otherwise, by the American Heart Association.

Organizations

The organizations listed below provide information and educational materials for people who are interested in keeping their hearts and cardiovascular systems in top running condition.

GENERAL INFORMATION

American Heart Association National Center
7272 Greenville Avenue
Dallas, TX 75231–4596
(800) AHA-USA-1
(See list of AHA Affiliates, pages 386–388.)

National Health Information Center
Office of Disease Prevention and Health Promotion
U.S. Public Health Service
Department of Health and Human Services
P.O. Box 1133
Washington, DC 20013–1133
(800) 336–4757

National Heart, Lung and Blood Institute
NHLBI Information Center
P.O. Box 30105
Bethesda, MD 20824–0105
(301) 251–1222

DIET, PHYSICAL ACTIVITY, WEIGHT MANAGEMENT, SMOKING CESSATION, EMOTIONAL HEALTH, TREATMENT, AND REHABILITATION

American Cancer Society
1599 Clifton Road NE
Atlanta, GA 30329
(800) 227–2345

American Diabetes Association
1660 Duke Street
Alexandria, VA 22314
(800) ADA-DISC

American Dietetic Association
216 West Jackson Boulevard
Suite 800
Chicago, IL 60606–6995
(800) 366–1655

American Lung Association
1740 Broadway
New York, NY 10019–4374
(212) 315–8700

Mended Hearts
Affiliated with the American Heart Association
7272 Greenville Avenue
Dallas, TX 75231–4596
(214) 706–1442

National Mental Health Association
1021 Prince Street
Alexandria, VA 22314–2971
(703) 684–7722

President's Council on Physical Fitness and Sports
701 Pennsylvania Avenue NW
Suite 250
Washington, DC 20004
(202) 272–3424

Stroke Connection
A Service of the American Heart Association
7272 Greenville Avenue
Dallas, TX 75231–4596
(800) 553–6321

LOCAL RESOURCES

Local Health Departments

Books

The following books may be available from your local bookstore, library, or rehabilitation group. Some books may also be ordered directly from the publisher.

American College of Sports Medicine, *ACSM Fitness Book,* Champaign, IL: Leisure Press, 1992.

American Heart Association. *American Heart Association Brand Name Fat and Cholesterol Counter*. New York: Times Books, 1991.

Blair, Steven N., P.E.D. *Living With Exercise*. Dallas: American Health Publishing Company, 1991.

Brownell, Kelly D., Ph.D. *The LEARN Program for Weight Control*. Dallas: American Health Publishing Company, 1994.

Caplan, Lou, M.D., Dyken, Mark L., M.D., and Easton, J. Donald, M.D., *American Heart Association Family Guide to Stroke: Treatment, Recovery, and Prevention*. New York: Times Books, 1994.

Connor, Sonja L., M.S., R.D. and William E. Connor, M.D. *The New American Diet System*. New York: Simon and Schuster, 1991.

Grundy, Scott., M.D., Ph.D., and Mary Winston, Ed.D., R.D., eds. *American Heart Association Low-Fat, Low-Cholesterol Cookbook*. New York: Times Books, 1989.

Starke, Rodman D., M.D., and Mary Winston, Ed.D., R.D., eds. *American Heart Association Low-Salt Cookbook*. New York: Times Books, 1990.

Warshaw, Hope S., M.M.Sc., R.D. *The Restaurant Companion*. Chicago: Surrey Books, 1990.

Winston, Mary, Ed.D., R.D., ed. *American Heart Association Cookbook*. Fifth Edition. New York: Times Books, 1991.

Periodicals

The following periodicals may be available from your local bookstore, library, or rehabilitation group. They may also be ordered directly from the publisher.

Cooking Light. Published eight times a year by Southern Living Inc., 2100 Lakeshore Drive, Birmingham, AL, 35209.

Heart Beat. Published four times a year by Mended Hearts, 7272 Greenville Avenue, Dallas, TX, 75231–4596.

Stroke Connection. Published six times a year by the American Heart Association's Stroke Connection, 7272 Greenville Avenue, Dallas, TX, 75231–4596.

Videocassette Tapes

The following tapes may be available from your local American Heart Association, hospital, library, or rehabilitation group. Some may be ordered directly from the company or association listed.

Active Partnership for the Health of Your Heart (series), American Heart Association, Dallas, Texas, (800) AHA-USA1, 1990.

   #1—Understanding Coronary Heart Disease
   #2—Taking Control
   #3—Quitting Smoking
   #4—A Lifetime of Good Eating
   #5—Exercise for Life
   #6—Staying Cool: Managing Stress

Eating Healthy on a Budget, Cable News Network, Atlanta, Georgia, 800–799–7676, 1994.

Eating Healthy when Dining Out, Cable News Network, Atlanta, Georgia, 800–799–7676, 1994.

Eating Healthy for Weight Control, Cable News Network, Atlanta, Georgia, 800–799–7676, 1994.

A Firsthand Lesson in Secondhand Smoke, American Heart Association, Dallas, Texas, (800) AHA-USA1, 1993.

Heart of the World, Cable News Network, Atlanta, Georgia, 800–799–7676, 1994.

The Taste of Eating Healthy, Cable News Network, Atlanta, Georgia, 800–799–7676, 1994.

Witch's Brew—Secondhand Smoke in the Workplace, American Heart Association, Dallas, Texas, (800) AHA-USA1, 1993.

Women and Heart Disease. American Heart Association, Dallas, Texas, (800) AHA-USA1, 1989.

APPENDIX C

American Heart Association Affiliates

American Heart Association
National Center
Dallas, TX

AHA, Alabama Affiliate, Inc.
Birmingham, AL

AHA, Alaska Affiliate, Inc.
Anchorage, AK

AHA, Arizona Affiliate, Inc.
Phoenix, AZ

AHA, Arkansas Affiliate, Inc.
Little Rock, AR

AHA, California Affiliate, Inc.
Burlingame, CA

AHA of Metropolitan Chicago,
Inc.
Chicago, IL

AHA of Colorado/Wyoming,
Inc.
Denver, CO

AHA, Connecticut Affiliate,
Inc.
Wallingford, CT

AHA, Dakota Affiliate, Inc.
Jamestown, ND

AHA, Delaware Affiliate, Inc.
Newark, DE

AHA, Florida Affiliate, Inc.
St. Petersburg, FL

AHA, Georgia Affiliate, Inc.
Marietta, GA

AHA, Hawaii Affiliate, Inc.
Honolulu, HI

AHA of Idaho/Montana, Inc.
Boise, ID

AHA, Illinois Affiliate, Inc.
Springfield, IL

AHA, Indiana Affiliate, Inc.
Indianapolis, IN

AHA, Iowa Affiliate, Inc.
Des Moines, IA

AHA, Kansas Affiliate, Inc.
Topeka, KS

AHA, Kentucky Affiliate, Inc.
Louisville, KY

AHA, Greater Los Angeles
Affiliate, Inc.
Los Angeles, CA

AHA, Louisiana Affiliate, Inc.
Destrehan, LA

AHA, Maine Affiliate, Inc.
Augusta, ME

AHA, Maryland Affiliate, Inc.
Baltimore, MD

AHA, Massachusetts Affiliate,
Inc.
Framingham, MA

AHA of Michigan, Inc.
Lathrup Village, MI

AHA, Minnesota Affiliate, Inc.
Minneapolis, MN

AHA, Mississippi Affiliate, Inc.
Jackson, MS

AHA, Missouri Affiliate, Inc.
St. Louis, MO

AHA, Nation's Capital
Affiliate, Inc.
Washington, D.C.

AHA, Nebraska Affiliate, Inc.
Omaha, NE

AHA, Nevada Affiliate, Inc.
Las Vegas, NV

AHA, New Hampshire
Affiliate, Inc.
Manchester, NH

AHA, New Jersey Affiliate, Inc.
North Brunswick, NJ

AHA, New Mexico Affiliate,
Inc.
Albuquerque, NM

AHA, New York City Affiliate,
Inc.
New York, NY

AHA, New York State Affiliate,
Inc.
North Syracuse, NY

AHA, North Carolina Affiliate,
Inc.
Chapel Hill, NC

AHA, Northeast Ohio Affiliate,
Inc.
Cleveland, OH

AHA, Ohio Affiliate, Inc.
Columbus, OH

AHA, Oklahoma Affiliate, Inc.
Oklahoma City, OK

AHA, Oregon Affiliate, Inc.
Portland, OR

AHA, Pennsylvania Affiliate,
Inc.
Camp Hill, PA

Puerto Rico Heart Association,
Inc.
Hato Rey, Puerto Rico

AHA, Rhode Island Affiliate,
Inc.
Pawtucket, RI

AHA, South Carolina Affiliate,
Inc.
Columbia, SC

AHA, Southeastern
Pennsylvania Affiliate, Inc.
Conshohocken, PA

AHA, Tennessee Affiliate, Inc.
Nashville, TN

AHA, Texas Affiliate, Inc.
Austin, TX

AHA, Utah Affiliate, Inc.
Salt Lake City, UT

AHA, Vermont Affiliate, Inc.
Williston, VT

AHA, Virginia Affiliate, Inc.
Glen Allen, VA

AHA, Washington Affiliate, Inc.
Seattle, WA

AHA, West Virginia Affiliate,
  Inc.
Charleston, WV

AHA, Wisconsin Affiliate, Inc.
Milwaukee, WI

GLOSSARY

Aerobic Exercise—Physical activities strenuously performed so as to cause marked temporary increases in respiration and heart rate. These include dynamic exercises and large muscle group activities such as walking and running.

Angina Pectoris—Medical term for chest pain due to coronary heart disease. A condition in which the heart muscle doesn't receive enough blood, resulting in pain in the chest.

Angiogram—An X-ray picture of blood vessels or chambers of the heart that shows the course of a special fluid called a contrast medium or dye injected into the bloodstream.

Angioplasty—A procedure sometimes used to dilate (widen) narrowed arteries. A catheter with a deflated balloon on its tip is passed into the narrowed artery segment, the balloon inflated, and the narrowed segment widened.

Aorta—The large artery that receives blood from the heart's left ventricle and distributes it to the body.

Aortic Valve—The heart valve between the left ventricle and the aorta. It has three flaps, or cusps.

389

Arrhythmia (or Dysrhythmia)—An abnormal rhythm of the heart.

Arteriography—A testing procedure in which an X-ray opaque dye is injected into the bloodstream, and then pictures are taken and studied to see if the arteries are damaged.

Arterioles—Small, muscular branches of arteries. When they contract, they increase resistance to blood flow, and blood pressure in the arteries increases.

Artery—Any one of a series of blood vessels that carry blood from the heart to the various parts of the body. Arteries have thick, elastic walls that can expand as blood flows through them.

Atherosclerosis—A form of arteriosclerosis in which the inner layers of artery walls become thick and irregular due to deposits of fat, cholesterol, and other substances. This buildup is sometimes called "plaque." As the interior walls of arteries become lined with layers of these deposits, the arteries become narrowed, and the flow of blood through them is reduced.

Atrium—Either one of the two upper chambers of the heart in which blood collects before being passed to the ventricles.

Bacterial Endocarditis—A bacterial infection of the heart lining or valves. People with abnormal heart valves or congenital heart defects are at increased risk of developing this disease.

Blood Clot—A jelly-like mass of blood tissue formed by clotting factors in the blood. This clot can then stop the flow of blood from an injury. Blood clots also can form inside an artery whose walls are damaged by atherosclerotic buildup and can cause a heart attack or stroke.

Blood Pressure—The force or pressure exerted by the heart in pumping blood; the pressure of blood in the arteries.

Calorie—A unit of measure that represents the amount of energy that is in foods. The term is also used to represent the amount of energy used by the body for basic body functions and the amount of energy expended through physical activity.

Capillaries—Microscopically small blood vessels between arteries and veins that distribute oxygenated blood to the body's tissues.

Cardiac—Pertaining to the heart.

Cardiac Arrest—The stopping of the heartbeat, usually because of interference with the electrical signal (often associated with coronary heart disease).

Cardiology—The study of the heart and its functions in health and disease.

Cardiomyopathy—A serious disease frequently affecting young people; it involves an inflammation and decreased function in heart muscle. There may be multiple causes including viral infections.

Cardiopulmonary Resuscitation (CPR)—A combination of chest compression and mouth-to-mouth breathing, this technique is used during cardiac arrest to keep oxygenated blood flowing to the heart muscle and brain until advanced cardiac life support can be started or an adequate heartbeat resumes.

Cardiovascular—Pertaining to the heart and blood vessels. ("Cardio" means heart; "vascular" means blood vessels.) The circulatory system of the heart and blood vessels is the cardiovascular system.

Carotid Artery—A major artery in the neck.

Catheterization—The process of examining the heart by introducing a thin tube (catheter) into a vein or artery and passing it into the heart.

Cholesterol—A fat-like substance found in animal tissue and present only in foods from animal sources such as whole milk dairy products, meat, fish, poultry, animal fats, and egg yolks.

Circulatory System—Pertaining to the heart, blood vessels, and the circulation of the blood.

Congenital—Refers to conditions existing at birth.

Congenital Heart Defects—Malformation of the heart or of its major blood vessels present at birth.

Congestive Heart Failure—The inability of the heart to pump out all the blood that returns to it. This results in blood backing up in the veins that lead to the heart and sometimes in fluid accumulating in various parts of the body.

Coronary Arteries—Two arteries arising from the aorta that arch down over the top of the heart, branch, and provide blood to the heart muscle.

Coronary Artery Disease—Conditions that cause narrowing of the coronary arteries so blood flow to the heart muscle is reduced.

Coronary Bypass Surgery—Surgery to improve blood supply to the heart muscle. This surgery is most often performed when narrowed coronary arteries reduce the flow of oxygen-containing blood to the heart itself.

Coronary Care Unit—A specialized facility in a hospital or emergency mobile unit that's equipped with monitoring devices and staffed with trained personnel. It's designed specifically to treat coronary patients.

Coronary Heart Disease—Disease of the heart caused by atherosclerotic narrowing of the coronary arteries likely to produce angina pectoris or heart attack; a general term.

Coronary Thrombosis—Formation of a clot in one of the arteries that conduct blood to the heart muscle. Also called coronary occlusion.

Defibrillator—An electronic device that helps reestablish normal contraction rhythms in a malfunctioning heart.

Diabetes—A disease in which the body doesn't produce or properly use insulin. Insulin is needed to convert sugar and starch into the energy needed in daily life. The full name for this condition is diabetes mellitus.

Diuretic—A drug that increases the rate at which urine forms by promoting the excretion of water and salts.

Echocardiography—A diagnostic method in which pulses of sound are transmitted into the body and the echoes returning from the surfaces of the heart and other structures are electronically plotted and recorded to produce a "picture" of the heart's size, shape, and movements.

Electrocardiogram (ECG or EKG)—A graphic record of electrical impulses produced by the heart.

Enzyme—A complex chemical capable of speeding up specific biochemical processes in the body.

Estrogen Replacement Therapy (ERT)—A therapuetic method that has been shown by large population studies to be beneficial in reducing the risk of coronary heart disease and osteoporosis.

Heart Attack—Death of, or damage to part of the heart muscle due to an insufficient blood supply.

Heart-Lung Machine—An apparatus that oxygenates and pumps blood to the body while a person's heart is opened for surgery.

Heredity—The genetic transmission of a particular quality or trait from parent to offspring.

High Blood Pressure—A chronic increase in blood pressure above its normal range.

High Density Lipoprotein (HDL)—A carrier of cholesterol believed to transport cholesterol away from the tissues and to the liver, where it can be removed from the bloodstream.

Hypertension—Same as High Blood Pressure.

Incidence—The number of new and recurrent cases of a disease that develops in a population during a specified period of time, such as a year.

Ischemia—Decreased blood flow to an organ, usually due to constriction or obstruction of an artery.

Kawasaki Disease—An acute children's illness of unknown cause that's characterized by fever, rash, swelling, and inflammation of various parts of the body. The coronary arteries or other parts of the heart are affected in up to 20 percent of children with this disease.

Lipoprotein—The combination of lipid surrounded by a protein; the protein makes it soluble in blood.

Low Density Lipoprotein (LDL)—The main carrier of "harmful" cholesterol in the blood.

Monounsaturated Fat—A type of fat found in many foods but predominantly in canola, olive, and peanut oil and avocados.

Myocardial Ischemia—Deficient blood flow to part of the heart muscle.

Myocardium—The muscular wall of the heart. It contracts to pump blood out of the heart and then relaxes as the heart refills with returning blood.

Obesity—The condition of being significantly overweight. It's usually applied to a condition of 20 percent or more over ideal body weight. Obesity puts a strain on the heart and can increase the chance of developing high blood pressure and diabetes.

Open Heart Surgery—Surgery performed on the opened heart while the bloodstream is diverted through a heart-lung machine.

Pacemaker—The "natural" pacemaker of the heart is called the sinus node. It's a small group of specialized cells in the top of the right atrium of the heart. It produces the electrical impulses that travel down to eventually reach the ventricular muscle, causing the heart to contract. The term "artificial pacemaker" is applied to an electrical device that can substitute for a defective natural pacemaker or conduction pathway. The artificial pacemaker controls the heart's beating by emitting a series of rhythmic electrical discharges.

Plaque—Also called atheroma, this is a deposit of fatty (and other) substances in the inner lining of the artery wall characteristic of atherosclerosis.

Polyunsaturated Fats—Oils of vegetable origin such as corn, safflower, sunflower, and soybean oil that are liquid at room temperature.

Premature ventricular contraction (PVC)—Irregular heartbeat that starts in the ventricles.

Pulmonary—Pertaining to the lungs.

Rheumatic Heart Disease—Damage done to the heart, particularly the heart valves, by one or more attacks of rheumatic fever.

Risk Factor—An element or condition involving certain hazard or danger. When referring to the heart and blood vessels, a risk factor is associated with an increased chance of developing cardiovascular disease including stroke.

Saturated Fats—Types of fat found in foods of animal origin and a few of vegetable origin; they are typically solid at room temperature.

Sedentary—Engages in minimal or no physical activity.

Silent Ischemia—Episodes of ischemia that aren't accompanied by pain.

Sodium—A mineral essential to life found in nearly all plant and animal tissue. Table salt (sodium chloride) is nearly half sodium.

Stress—Bodily or mental tension within a person resulting from his or her response to physical, chemical, or emotional factors. Stress can refer to physical exertion as well as mental anxiety.

Stroke (also called Apoplexy, Cerebrovascular Accident, or Cerebral Vascular Accident)—Loss of muscle function, vision, sensation, or speech resulting from brain cell damage caused by an insufficient supply of blood to part of the brain.

Sudden Cardiac Death—Death that occurs unexpectedly and instantaneously or shortly after the onset of symptoms. The most common underlying reason for patients dying suddenly is cardiovascular disease, in particular coronary heart disease.

Systolic Blood Pressure—The highest blood pressure measured in the arteries. It occurs when the heart contracts with each heartbeat.

Thallium Scan—A medical diagnostic test in which thallium, a radioactive isotope, is injected in a vein during exercise and then scanned with a special instrument in an effort to detect myocardial ischemia.

Thrombosis—The formation or presence of a blood clot (thrombus) inside a blood vessel or cavity of the heart.

Transient Ischemic Attack (TIA)—A temporary stroke-like event that lasts for only a short time and is caused by a temporarily blocked blood vessel.

Triglyceride—A fat that comes from food or is made in the body from other energy sources such as carbohydrates.

Ultrasound—High-frequency sound vibrations, not audible to the human ear, used in medical diagnosis.

Vascular—Pertaining to blood vessels.

Vein—Any one of a series of blood vessels of the vascular system that carries blood from various parts of the body back to the heart.

Ventricle—One of the two lower chambers of the heart.

INDEX

399

400